MASTERING PATHOPHYSIOLOGY: FUNDAMENTALS OF DISEASE AND TREATMENT, THE ESSENTIAL GUIDE TO TREATING THE MOST COMMON ILLNESSES AND CONDITIONS.

D. Beck

I Want to thank you and congratulate you for buying my book
Mastering Pathophysiology

CONTENTS

INTRODUCTION

Pathophysiology is the scientific study of the disordered physiological processes associated with disease or injury. It includes both structural and functional changes in organs, tissues, and cells that can lead to a wide range of clinical symptoms or signs in an individual. Pathophysiology is used to better understand how diseases progress and develop treatment plans for sufferers. By understanding the processes of disease, clinicians can provide more effective treatments for patients.

Pathophysiology is a broad field that encompasses many different areas such as cellular pathways, biochemical networks, genetic mutations, and immunological disorders. It also includes the impact of environmental factors on physiology. For example, studies have shown that air pollution can increase inflammation and cause damage to vital organs and tissues.

Pathophysiology also includes the study of psychological disorders, such as depression and anxiety. Research has shown that there are genetic and biochemical factors involved in these types of illnesses, which can affect an individual's overall health and quality of life. By understanding how psychological disorders develop and progress, clinicians can better diagnose individuals with these conditions and develop appropriate treatment plans.

In addition to its role in understanding and treating diseases, pathophysiology can also help identify potential risk factors for disease development. By analyzing the physiological processes involved in a particular illness, researchers can understand which environmental, lifestyle, or genetic factors may contribute to an individual's risk of developing the condition. This information can be used to design effective prevention strategies and tailor treatments to individual needs.

Pathophysiology is an invaluable tool for the medical community, as it helps to better understand how diseases progress and inform effective treatment plans. By studying pathophysiology, clinicians are able to provide more personalized care for their patients and improve overall health outcomes.

Hello, it's me, D.Beck . Before you start reading my book I would like to ask you a favor: If you enjoy reading the book can you please leave an honest review for me in Amazon? - it will mean a lot to me! Thanks in advantage, and now be ready to learn more about Pathophysiology :)

CHAPTER 1: WHAT IS PATHOPHYSIOLOGY?

Pathophysiology is the study of changes in bodily functions due to disease or injury. It deals with a wide range of disorders and diseases, from acute illnesses such as colds to chronic conditions such as cancer. Pathophysiologists analyze how these changes affect the body's response to illness or injury and also focus on possible methods of treatment and prevention.

Pathophysiology is an important field of medicine, as it can help doctors understand the underlying causes of disease and develop a treatment plan. By understanding how certain changes in bodily functions lead to diseases or injury, doctors are better able to diagnose and treat conditions. Pathophysiology also helps physicians understand how treatments may work on different types of patients.

Pathophysiology also helps researchers develop new treatments for various diseases. By studying the pathophysiology of a disease, researchers can better understand how it affects different people and how current treatments are working. In addition, research into pathophysiology can aid in the development of new medications or treatments that may be more effective at treating certain diseases than existing ones.

History Of Pathophysiology

Pathophysiology is a branch of medicine that focuses on the study of abnormal changes in body functions. It has a long history, with some of its earliest roots dating back to antiquity. Ancient Greek and Roman physicians were among the first to document how pathology affected the body. They also made significant contributions to our understanding of diseases such as leprosy, typhoid fever, smallpox, and rabies.

In the Middle Ages, many diseases were not understood. Physicians largely based their treatments on superstition and folklore. However, medical literature began to appear in the 16th century with publications from distinguished scholars such as Ambroise Pare and Paracelsus. These works provided insight into pathophysiology and helped advance its development.

The modern science of pathophysiology began in the 19th century with the development of new clinical techniques such as auscultation and percussion. German physician Rudolf Virchow is credited for formulating the cell theory, which serves as a major pillar of medicine today. In addition, British scientists Joseph Lister and Louis Pasteur introduced germ theory to further explain the cause of disease.

The 20th century saw remarkable advances in pathophysiology with the development and widespread use of antibiotics, vaccinations, and other drugs. These treatments revolutionized medicine and led to a greater understanding of how different diseases function at the cellular level.

Today, pathophysiology is an essential part of medical education. By applying their knowledge of anatomy, physiology, biochemistry, and other sciences, physicians can accurately identify and treat diseases. Pathophysiology continues to evolve as researchers make new discoveries about the body's functions and interactions with its environment.

Pathophysiology is a critical part of our medical landscape today. It provides clinicians with the tools they need to properly diagnose and effectively manage illnesses in order to improve patient outcomes. With its long and storied past, pathophysiology is an integral component of modern medicine.

Explain The Importance Of Studying Pathophysiology

Pathophysiology is the study of the changes in body functions and structures caused by disease. It allows us to understand how diseases develop, progress, and end. By studying pathophysiology we can identify how a certain disease or group of diseases affects our bodies and what treatment options are available. Additionally, it can help scientists better understand the underlying causes of certain conditions.

This knowledge is essential for healthcare providers to accurately diagnose and treat medical conditions. By providing a better understanding of the different components of a disease, healthcare providers can determine the best course of action to take in order to reduce symptoms and improve quality of life. Pathophysiology also gives researchers insight into how our bodies respond to certain treatments, allowing us to develop more effective therapies for chronic diseases and other medical conditions.

What Is The Importance Of Studying Pathophysiology?

1. Pathophysiology is a crucial area of medical study as it helps to understand how the disease affects the body at a cellular level. This knowledge can be used to develop treatments that target specific areas of the body and provide relief for patients.
2. By studying pathophysiology, medical professionals are able to gain an understanding of diseases, their symptoms, and how they affect the overall functioning of the body. This

knowledge can be used to develop strategies for diagnosis, treatment, and prevention of disease.

3. Pathophysiology is also important for medical researchers as it helps them to better understand how different diseases interact with each other and how their symptoms manifest in patients. Understanding this complex relationship between diseases and treatments allows researchers to create more effective treatments for patients.

4. Pathophysiology is also essential for medical students as it provides them with an understanding of how the body functions and how it responds to different stimuli. This knowledge can be used to develop a greater understanding of disease and allow them to provide better patient care.

5. pathophysiology helps clinicians to further their knowledge of diseases and the treatments available. This can help them to make informed decisions about how to treat their patients and provide effective, safe care for them. By understanding the underlying causes of disease, they can better tailor treatments to their individual needs.

What Are The Basics Of Pathophysiology?

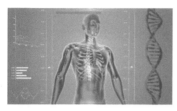 Pathophysiology is a branch of medicine that studies the changes in a person's body due to disease or injury. It looks at how the body responds to these changes and how it tries to maintain normal function. Pathophysiologists look at the cause, progression, signs and symptoms, diagnosis, treatment, and long-term outcomes of illnesses or injuries.

Pathophysiology focuses on the body as a whole and its interactions with other physiological systems. It examines the anatomy, biochemistry, and physiology of cells, tissues, organs, and organ systems to understand how diseases or injuries affect normal functioning.

The foundations of pathophysiology include understanding abnormal processes such as inflammation, infection, neoplasia (abnormal tissue growth), and the body's response to trauma or stress. Pathophysiology also looks at how genetic mutations, environmental factors, and lifestyle choices can alter a person's physiology, leading to an abnormal condition.

Pathophysiology plays an important role in medical research by helping scientists identify new treatments for diseases and injuries. It is also helpful in determining why some treatments work better than others for certain conditions.

Ultimately, understanding the pathophysiology of a particular disease or injury can help doctors provide more effective care to their patients.

Pathophysiology is an ever-evolving field that is constantly developing new ways to diagnose and treat illnesses and injuries. It involves a complex web of interactions between many different physiological systems, so it is a field that requires years of study and experience to understand fully.

Who Is A Pathophysiologist?

Pathophysiology is the medical sub-speciality that focuses on how diseases and conditions affect the human body. Pathophysiologists use their knowledge and expertise to analyze the changes in normal bodily functions due to illness or injury. They assess the effects of illnesses and other health conditions on a person's physical, psychological, behavioural, and social well-being. As such, they make diagnoses, develop treatment plans, and provide care to patients.

Pathophysiologists are integral members of the healthcare team and may work in private medical practices, hospitals, clinics, public health departments, universities, research laboratories or other settings. Depending on their specialization level and backgrounds, a pathophysiologist's duties may include managing patients with disease-related conditions, conducting research studies on the causes of disease and disability, developing new treatments or therapies for chronic illnesses, consulting with other healthcare professionals to provide quality care, teaching students about diseases and their prevention, creating health promotion campaigns and interventions, and managing clinical trials.

The pathophysiologist requires an extensive knowledge base in many scientific disciplines including anatomy and physiology; pathology; nutrition; pharmacology; and epidemiology. They must also have a firm grasp of the principles of medicine, surgery, public health, and medical law. A successful pathophysiologist is able to assess patients efficiently and accurately diagnose diseases by identifying symptoms and performing diagnostic tests.

Pathophysiologists work closely with other healthcare professionals to identify treatments that are in the best interest of the patient. They employ a range of treatments including medication, surgery, lifestyle changes, and supplements to help patients manage their conditions. Pathologists also work to evaluate new medications or therapies prior to introducing them into practice. By doing so, they can ensure that potential treatments are safe and effective for patients.

The career outlook for pathophysiologists is encouraging. As the population ages, there will be an increase in healthcare demands and more need for qualified pathophysiologists to help meet those needs. Pathophysiology offers a chance for professionals to make a meaningful impact on patient care. With the right qualifications and training, anyone can become successful in this field.

Terminologies In Pathophysiology

There are several terms used in pathophysiology to describe certain conditions and diseases. Some of these terminologies include:

Acute:

A medical term used to describe the onset of a disease or symptom that is rapid and severe. An acute condition typically has a short duration, but can sometimes become chronic if not treated.

Collection:

The accumulation of fluid, cells, or other materials in a localized area of the body due to inflammation or injury. Collections can be an indication of infection and require medical attention.

Systemic:

A term used to describe a disease or condition that affects the entire body. Systemic disorders can have many symptoms and require a comprehensive medical approach to diagnose and manage.

Pathology:

The study of disease or injury, including the changes in tissues caused by the disease or injury. Pathology is an important field because it helps doctors understand how diseases develop and how to treat them effectively.

Pathogenesis:

The process by which a disease or condition develops and progresses. Pathogenesis is used to understand the progression of a specific disorder and how it can be best managed.

Symptomology:

The study of symptoms and signs associated with a disease or condition. Symptomology helps doctors recognize diseases before they become more serious and can be used to track the progression of a disorder over time.

These terminologies are important for understanding pathophysiology, and how diseases and conditions develop. Knowing these terms can help physicians diagnose and treat their patients effectively.

CHAPTER 2: KEY CONCEPTS
OF PATHOPHYSIOLOGY :

1. Homeostasis

Homeostasis is the process by which organisms maintain a stable internal environment. This means that the organism manages to keep its internal conditions (such as temperature, pH, and other parameters) within an acceptable range despite changes in the external environment. Homeostasis is a vital concept in pathophysiology because it helps us understand how the disease affects our body's ability to maintain normal functioning.

For example, diabetes is a condition where the body cannot properly regulate its blood glucose levels. In this case, the homeostatic mechanisms are not working correctly and the patient needs some external help (e.g., insulin injections) in order to keep their glucose levels within an acceptable range. Similarly, in hypertension, the body is unable to maintain normal blood pressure due to faulty mechanisms of homeostasis.

The concept of homeostasis can also be applied to other physiological processes such as respiration and digestion. In respiratory disorders (e.g., asthma), the body's ability to regulate breathing is impaired, leading to shortness of breath and difficulty in breathing. In digestive disorders (e.g., Crohn's disease), the body is unable to regulate digestion and absorption, leading to a variety of symptoms such as abdominal pain, weight loss, and diarrhoea.

By understanding the concept of homeostasis, we can gain a better understanding of how diseases affect our bodies and what treatments may be available to help restore balance and normal functioning. Homeostasis is a fundamental concept in the study of pathophysiology, and any healthcare professional needs to understand its implications.

What Are The Implications Of Homeostasis For Pathophysiology?

The implications of homeostasis for pathophysiology are critical, as knowing how the body maintains balance in its internal environment can help us to better diagnose and treat diseases. By understanding how homeostatic processes fail, we can discern what treatments and therapies are necessary to restore balance and health.

For example, a patient with diabetes has difficulty maintaining their blood glucose levels within an acceptable range. In this case, knowing how the body normally regulates glucose levels can help us to identify what treatments are necessary and how to adjust the patient's diet. Similarly, understanding the process of homeostasis in respiration and digestion can help us to better treat pulmonary diseases such as asthma or digestive disorders such as Crohn's disease.

2. Pathogenesis

Pathogenesis is the process by which a disease develops. It involves four elements: the agent (e.g., virus or bacteria), the host (the organism in which the disease occurs), the environment, and any factors that can influence pathogenesis (such as genetics). Pathogenesis includes all of the processes related to how a particular disease develops, such as how it is transmitted, its symptoms, and the potential treatments and therapies for managing it. Pathogenesis is an important concept to understand in pathophysiology, as it helps us to identify how diseases develop and progress so that we can provide better care for our patients. Understanding pathogenesis can also help us to develop more effective preventative measures for a particular disease.

Pathogenesis is closely related to homeostasis in that the failure of the body's normal processes can lead to a disruption in homeostasis, which then leads to disease. For example, a virus or bacteria invading the body can disrupt homeostatic mechanisms and cause inflammation, which can then lead to disease. Pathogenesis also involves how our environment affects our health; for instance, exposure to certain environmental toxins can weaken our immune system, making us more susceptible to disease.

By understanding pathogenesis, we can gain a better understanding of how diseases develop and progress and how we can prevent or treat them. Pathogenesis is an important concept in the study of pathophysiology, as it helps us to identify the underlying causes of disease and provide better care for our patients.

What Are The Implications Of Pathogenesis For Pathophysiology?

The implications of pathogenesis for pathophysiology are far-reaching. Knowing the underlying causes of a disease can help us more accurately diagnose and treat it, as well as develop better preventative measures. Pathogenesis also helps us to identify risk factors that may put certain individuals at greater risk for a particular disease. For example, exposure to environmental toxins such as air pollution or certain chemicals can increase the risk of developing a respiratory disorder or other illnesses.

Pathogenesis is also closely related to homeostasis, as the disruption of homeostatic processes can lead to disease. By understanding how our environment and genetic makeup can influence pathogenesis, we can gain a better understanding of how diseases develop and progress and what treatments may be necessary.

3. Etiology

Etiology is the study of the causes of a particular disease. In pathophysiology, etiology involves identifying what processes and factors lead to a particular disease. Etiological studies are important for helping us understand how diseases develop and progress so that we can provide better care for our patients.

Common factors that may contribute to the etiology of the disease include environmental factors such as air pollution, genetic predispositions, lifestyle factors such as diet and smoking, and infectious agents such as bacteria or viruses. Additionally, etiology may involve studying how a particular disease affects different populations (e.g., racial disparities in certain illnesses) or identifying the underlying biological mechanisms that cause disease.

Etiology can also help us to identify risk factors for a particular disease. For example, lifestyle choices such as smoking or diet can be identified as potential risk factors for developing certain diseases. By understanding the etiology of a disease, we can gain a better understanding of how to prevent it and how to treat it more effectively.

What Are The Implications Of Etiology For

Pathophysiology?

The implications of etiology for pathophysiology are significant. Knowing the causes of a particular disease can help us to better diagnose and treat it, as well as develop preventative measures. By identifying environmental and lifestyle factors that may contribute to the development of a disease, we can gain a better understanding of how to reduce its incidence in the population.

Etiology can also help us to identify risk factors that may put certain individuals at greater risk for a particular disease. For example, individuals with a family history of a particular illness or those who are exposed to environmental toxins may be more likely to develop the disease than others.

By understanding etiology, we can gain insight into how diseases develop and progress, what treatments may be necessary, and how to more effectively manage them. Etiology is an important concept in the study of pathophysiology, as it helps us to identify the underlying causes of disease and provide better care for our patients.

What Are Some Examples Of Etiological Studies?

Examples of etiological studies include epidemiological studies, which examine the causes and patterns of diseases in a population; clinical studies, which test treatments and therapies; molecular genetic studies, which identify risk factors associated with a particular disease; and environmental studies, which look at the role of environment in disease development.

Etiology can also involve social and behavioural studies to understand how lifestyle choices, such as diet and exercise, can influence disease development. Additionally, etiological studies can involve the study of infectious agents to identify which pathogens may be responsible for a particular illness.

4. Morbidity

Morbidity is an important concept in the study of pathophysiology, as it helps us to understand how a particular disease affects individuals and populations. Morbidity refers to the frequency or number of cases of a particular disease in a population. It can also refer to the severity or degree of illness associated with a particular disease.

For example, the morbidity of a particular disease can be measured by the number of cases (incidence) or the number of deaths (mortality). Additionally, morbidity may also involve looking at other factors such as hospitalizations, disability rates, and quality of life.

Morbidity can help us to identify trends in a population and to understand how a particular disease affects individuals. It can also be used to compare the prevalence of a disease in different populations and to measure the health burden associated with a particular illness.

By understanding morbidity, we can gain insight into how diseases affect different populations and develop better treatments or prevention measures. Morbidity is an important concept in pathophysiology, as it gives us a better understanding of the impact of a particular disease on individuals and populations.

For instance, by understanding morbidity, we can identify trends in the prevalence of various diseases across different populations. This may help us to develop targeted prevention measures or treatments for certain illnesses, as well as identify risk factors that increase an individual's likelihood of developing a particular illness. Additionally, knowing the morbidity of a particular disease can help us to understand the health burden associated with it and develop more effective ways to manage or treat it.

5. Prognosis

Prognosis is an important concept in the study of pathophysiology. Prognosis refers to the likely outcome or course of a particular disease, and it is used to predict how an illness will progress over time. By understanding prognosis, we can gain insight into what treatments may be necessary for a particular patient and determine what steps should be taken to improve their health outcomes.

For example, prognosis can help us to identify the most effective treatments for a particular illness or determine whether a patient is likely to require long-term care. Additionally, prognosis can also be used to predict how an individual's condition may progress and what kinds of complications they may develop over time.

Knowing the prognosis of a particular illness can help us to effectively plan and manage treatments, as well as identify risk factors that may influence the course of an individual's disease. Additionally, prognosis can provide valuable insight into how certain therapies may affect a patient's progress or how their condition may change over time.

Understanding prognosis is an important part of pathophysiology, as it helps us to identify the most effective treatments and management strategies for a particular disease. By understanding prognosis, we can gain insight into how a particular illness may progress and develop targeted interventions that will improve patient outcomes.

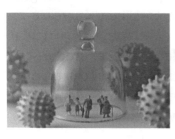

6. Epidemiology

Epidemiology is a branch of public health that focuses on the study of patterns and causes of diseases in populations. It involves looking at factors such as environmental exposures, lifestyle choices, and genetic predispositions to understand how they affect disease development. Epidemiological studies can help us to understand how particular diseases spread in a population, what risk factors are associated with them, and how to prevent or manage them.

By understanding epidemiology, we can gain insight into how diseases develop and progress, as well as identify risk factors that may increase an individual's likelihood of developing a particular illness. Additionally, epidemiological studies can help us to understand the health burden associated with various illnesses and to develop better treatments or prevention measures.

What Are The Implications Of Epidemiology For Pathophysiology?

The study of epidemiology has significant implications for pathophysiology, as it can help us to better understand how diseases develop and progress. By studying the patterns and causes of diseases in a population, we can gain insight into what risk factors may increase an individual's likelihood of developing a particular illness. Additionally, epidemiological studies can provide valuable information on how to prevent or manage particular illnesses, as well as identify the health burden associated with them.

By understanding epidemiology, we can also

gain insight into how certain treatments may affect a patient's progress or what kind of complications they may develop over time. Additionally, epidemiological studies can provide valuable information on how to develop targeted interventions that will improve patient outcomes.

7. Comorbidity

Comorbidity is a term used to describe two or more chronic medical conditions that co-exist in one person. It typically occurs when a person has both physical and mental health issues, although it can also involve different physical illnesses. For example, someone with diabetes may also have high blood pressure, depression, anxiety, or other associated conditions. The effects of comorbidity can be significant, as it can make managing symptoms of both illnesses more difficult. Treatment plans may also need to be adjusted in order to address multiple conditions simultaneously. It is important to recognize and manage the implications of comorbidity in order to ensure that individuals receive the best possible care for their medical issues.

Comorbidity may also occur when a person has a combination of physical health conditions, such as diabetes and cardiovascular disease. In this case, the individual may have an increased risk of developing complications due to the associated comorbidities, such as kidney failure or stroke.

Additionally, comorbidity can lead to additional difficulties in managing symptoms, such as impaired mobility or difficulty performing basic activities of daily living. Healthcare providers need to be aware of the potential risks associated with comorbidity and take steps to mitigate them, such as providing adequate education about managing multiple conditions or referring patients to specialists when necessary.

Comorbidity can also have an effect on overall quality of life, reducing a person's ability to participate in activities they enjoy or leave them feeling overwhelmed and isolated. Healthcare providers need to recognize the potential emotional impacts that comorbidity can have on individuals and provide appropriate resources to support their mental health. This could involve referrals to mental health specialists, offering psychoeducation about managing multiple conditions, or providing access to online self-management tools.

What Are The Implications Of Comorbidity For Pathophysiology?

Comorbidity can significantly influence the pathophysiology of an illness, as it often affects how treatment plans should be structured and implemented. For example, a person with both diabetes and hypertension may need to take medications for both conditions, but their dosages and frequencies could differ greatly from someone who only has one condition. In addition, comorbidity can also lead to changes in the course of an illness, as different conditions may interact with each other or cause new symptoms. Therefore, healthcare providers need to take comorbidity into account when making decisions and developing treatment plans.

Comorbidity can also have a major impact on the clinical outcomes of a condition. For example, someone with both diabetes and hypertension may be more likely to experience complications such as stroke or kidney failure, even if their conditions are well managed. Additionally, comorbidity can add a layer of complexity to the diagnosis process, as symptoms of one condition could be caused by another or vice versa. Therefore, healthcare providers must consider the implications of comorbidity when diagnosing and managing medical conditions.

Finally, comorbidity can also have a major effect on the health-related quality of life (HRQOL) of individuals with chronic illnesses. A person with multiple conditions may experience increased levels of disability or difficulty performing activities of daily living due to their comorbidities, leading to reduced HRQOL. Therefore, healthcare providers must be aware of the effect comorbidity can have on individuals and provide appropriate resources and support to help manage their chronic conditions.

8. Syndromes

Syndromes are a group of signs and symptoms that occur together and characterize a particular abnormality or condition. They can be caused by either genetic factors, environmental influences, or a combination of both. A syndrome may also include physical findings, such as the presence of certain birth defects or anatomical abnormalities like microcephaly. Examples of syndromes include Down Syndrome, Turner Syndrome, Klinefelter Syndrome, and Fragile X Syndrome.

Many syndromes are associated with an underlying genetic cause, such as a chromosomal abnormality or a gene mutation. Syndromes can also have environmental causes, like exposure to certain substances during pregnancy. In some cases, the syndrome is caused by both genetics and the environment.

Syndromes can be divided into two main types: syndromes with recognizable physical features, and syndromes without recognizable physical features. Syndromes with recognizable physical features include Down Syndrome, Turner Syndrome, and Klinefelter Syndrome. Syndromes without recognizable physical features include Fragile X Syndrome, Rett Syndrome, Angelman Syndrome, and Prader-Willi Syndrome.

The diagnosis of a syndrome is based

on the recognition of certain clinical signs and symptoms, such as physical features or developmental delays. Diagnostic tests, such as chromosomal analysis or genetic testing, may also be used to confirm the diagnosis. Treatment and management of syndromes varies depending on the type and severity of the syndrome. Treatment and management may include physical, occupational, and/or speech therapy, as well as behavioural interventions. Some syndromes may also respond to specific medications or dietary changes.

It is important to understand that each individual with a syndrome is unique and the effects of the syndrome can range from mild to severe. With proper care and support, individuals with syndromes can lead productive and fulfilling lives.

In addition to medical management, individuals with syndromes may benefit from psychosocial support. This includes providing emotional support, giving informational resources, helping families find appropriate educational and recreational programs, and connecting them with other families who have similar experiences. Such support can help individuals with syndromes lead more meaningful lives and become more successful in their daily activities.

It is also important for healthcare providers to be familiar with common syndromes, as they can often help identify signs and symptoms that should be monitored or evaluated further. This knowledge can help physicians provide the best possible care for their patients.

What Are The Implications Of Syndromes For Pathophysiology?

The implications of syndromes for pathophysiology are vast and varied. Syndromes can provide insight into how underlying genetic and environmental factors interact to cause a disease or disorder. Understanding the molecular basis of these interactions can help physicians accurately diagnose, effectively treat, and potentially prevent certain disorders associated with syndromes.

In addition, understanding how different syndromes can affect pathways in the body can help physicians determine which treatments are appropriate for a particular individual. For example, this knowledge may impact decisions about the type of medication to prescribe or the lifestyle modifications that should be recommended.

Finally, research into syndromes may provide insight into how other diseases and conditions develop. Studying these syndromes can teach us more about the underlying causes of a wide variety of diseases and disorders, which can lead to improved treatment options and better outcomes for patients.

Ultimately, syndromes are complex yet fascinating topics that have significant implications for pathophysiology. Through research and collaboration, we can continue to learn more about how syndromes affect our health and work towards improving the lives of those affected.

9. Pharmacotherapy

Pharmacotherapy, also known as medication therapy, is the use of medications to treat various diseases and conditions. Through this approach, certain drugs can be used to reduce the symptoms of a disease or condition or even halt its progression. In order for these therapeutic effects to occur, pharmacotherapy must follow specific protocols in dosing, timing, and safety considerations. In addition, pharmacotherapy must be used in conjunction with non-pharmacological therapies such as lifestyle modifications and patient education to help improve the overall health of a patient.

There are several different types of medications available for patients, depending on their condition and needs. Commonly prescribed medications include anticonvulsants, antidepressants, anxiolytics, antipsychotics, diuretics, antihypertensive blockers, and immunosuppressants. It is important to note that while pharmacotherapy can be beneficial in treating a disease or condition, it also carries certain risks. Adverse drug reactions are common with medications and should be monitored closely by the healthcare team to ensure proper treatment and safety of the patient.

In addition to pharmacotherapy, complementary and alternative medicine (CAM) therapies may also be used to treat certain diseases or conditions. Examples of CAM therapies include acupuncture, herbal remedies, yoga, meditation, massage therapy, and tai chi. While these forms of treatment are becoming more widely accepted by medical professionals and patients alike, it is important to discuss any CAM therapies with a qualified healthcare professional to ensure appropriate use and safety.

The risk-benefit ratio of pharmacotherapy should be carefully evaluated by the patient and their doctor before beginning any treatment plan. It is important to understand the potential risks involved in taking medications and weigh them against the benefits that they may provide. With careful evaluation and monitoring, pharmacotherapy can be an effective way to manage and treat many diseases and conditions.

What Are The Implications Of Pharmacotherapy For Pathophysiology?

The use of pharmacotherapy in treating various diseases and conditions is an important part of pathophysiology. By understanding how different drugs work and interact with the human body, healthcare professionals are able to develop more effective treatments for a wide range of diseases and conditions. Pharmacological therapies allow for better symptom relief, halting or slowing the progression of certain diseases, and even helping to improve the overall health of patients.

While pharmacotherapy can be an effective way to treat many diseases and conditions, it is important to consider the potential risks that come along with taking medications. Adverse drug reactions are common and should be monitored closely by the patient's healthcare team. In addition, it is important to weigh the risk-benefit ratio of any pharmacological therapies before beginning a treatment plan.

When used appropriately and in concert with non-pharmacological therapies, pharmacotherapy can be an effective tool in treating and managing many diseases and conditions. It is important to discuss any concerns or questions with a qualified healthcare professional prior to beginning any treatments.

CHAPTER 3: BODY SYSTEMS

H ematologic system
The hematologic system is responsible for the production, maintenance, and flow of cells in the blood. This includes red blood cells (RBCs), white blood cells (WBCs), platelets, and plasma. The term "hematology" comes from two Greek words – hema meaning "blood" and logos meaning "science".

The normal range of RBCs is usually between 4.5 million and 5.5 million per cubic millimetre (mm³). They are responsible for carrying oxygen through the body and removing carbon dioxide from the cells. The normal range of WBCs is typically between 5,000 and 10,000 per mm³. These cells play an important role in the body's immune response to infection and foreign substances. Platelets are also a type of cell, though they do not contain nuclei like other blood cells. They are essential for clotting and help repair damaged tissue.

The plasma is a liquid component of the blood which contains proteins, electrolytes, and other substances. It helps to transport nutrients, hormones, and enzymes throughout the body. When the number of RBCs or WBCs is either too high or too low in comparison to normal ranges, it can be indicative of an underlying disease or disorder. Additionally, abnormal levels of plasma proteins can signal a variety of conditions, including kidney failure and cancer.

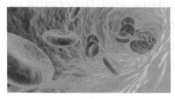

Understanding The Basis Of Hematologic System Diseases

Hematologic system diseases can also help us to better understand how diseases progress and what measures we can take to reduce their severity or even prevent them from developing in the first place. For example, some hematologic system diseases, such as sickle cell anaemia, are caused by genetic mutations that can be prevented through genetic counseling and early diagnosis. Other diseases, such as leukemia, may have environmental or lifestyle factors that contribute to their development. By understanding the role of these factors, we can take steps to reduce our risk of developing these illnesses.

Ultimately, pathophysiology plays an important role in helping us better understand hematologic system diseases and determine which treatments may be most effective for each individual patient. By understanding how different diseases develop and progress, physicians can better tailor treatment plans to each patient's unique needs and help them find the best possible outcome.

Role Of Pathophysiology In Hematologic System Diseases Development

Pathophysiology is the study of how diseases or injuries affect the structure and functions of different tissues, organs and cells in our body. This is important to understand because it provides insights into both how we can better diagnose a disease as well as inform us on how to treat that particular illness. In terms of hematologic system diseases, pathophysiology helps doctors and other medical professionals to better understand the signs and symptoms of these diseases, how they develop, and how to treat or prevent them.

The hematologic system is responsible for producing blood cells that are essential for our body's functioning. These include white blood cells (which protect us from infection), red blood cells (which transport oxygen throughout the body), platelets (which help with clotting) and other cell types. Diseases of the hematologic system can be caused by a variety of factors, such as genetic mutations, environmental exposure, or certain medications.

When it comes to understanding the pathophysiology of hematologic system diseases, there are a few key concepts that physicians must be aware of in order to identify and treat these illnesses. One important concept is the role of inflammation in hematologic system diseases. Inflammation occurs when the body's immune system identifies a foreign substance or invaders, such as viruses or bacteria, and responds by secreting chemicals that cause swelling and redness in the affected area. This response can be beneficial if it helps to fight off the invading organisms, but it can also have a negative effect when it causes damage to our own tissues and cells.

In addition, pathophysiology helps us to better understand how different medications and treatments for hematologic system diseases work. For example, some drugs help to reduce inflammation in order to decrease the severity of symptoms associated with various illnesses. Other drugs are designed to target specific cells, such as white blood cells, in order to reduce the number of these cells in the body or alter their function. By understanding how different treatments work, physicians can better tailor a treatment plan for each individual patient based on their diagnosis and symptoms.

Immune System

The immune system is a complex network of organs and cells that protect the body against foreign invaders. It is responsible for recognizing and eliminating harmful pathogens, such as viruses and bacteria, while also maintaining tolerance to non-harmful substances like food particles or pollen. The main components of the immune system include lymphoid tissue (such as the thymus, spleen, and lymph nodes), specialized white blood cells (such as B and T cells) and antibodies.

The immune system has two main lines of defense: the innate or nonspecific response, which is a quick but limited reaction to infection; and the adaptive or specific immunity which can develop over time in response to a particular type of pathogen. The adaptive response involves specific white blood cells, called B and T lymphocytes, which recognize antigens and produce antibodies that attack and eliminate the pathogen.

Immune system dysfunction can lead to disorders such as allergies, asthma, autoimmune diseases, and cancer. In these cases, the immune system has become hyperactive and begins to attack or overreact to harmless substances. To counteract this, immunosuppressant drugs can be used to suppress the immune system and reduce inflammation. In addition, certain lifestyle factors such as diet, exercise, and stress management can help maintain a healthy immune system.

Understanding The Basis Of Immune System Diseases

Researchers have identified several genes and pathways associated with the development of immune system disorders, but further research is needed to identify new therapeutic targets. In addition, there is increasing interest in using personalized medicine approaches to better diagnose and treat these conditions. By studying how individual patients' genetic makeup affects their response to treatment, doctors can tailor therapies that will be more effective for that patient.

Immune system diseases can also involve the dysfunction of other body systems, such as the nervous system and endocrine system. For instance, autoimmune disorders like multiple sclerosis or type 1 diabetes are caused by an attack on healthy tissues by the immune system. Thus, it is important to consider how all of these organ systems interact when treating patients with immune system disorders.

In recent years, researchers have developed new treatments that take advantage of the body's own natural healing abilities. For example, some therapies use antibodies or other proteins to block the activity of pro-inflammatory signals and reduce inflammation caused by autoimmune diseases. Additionally, stem cell therapy is being used to replace lost or damaged tissue in order to restore the function of certain organs.

Finally, there is an increasing focus on preventative measures for immune system diseases. These can include lifestyle changes such as improved diet and exercise, as well as immunizations to help protect against infectious diseases. By understanding the pathophysiology of these conditions, researchers can continue to develop new treatments and prevention strategies that will ultimately improve the lives of those affected by immune system disorders.

Role Of Pathophysiology In Immune System Diseases Development

Pathophysiology is the study of how diseases affect the body, particularly on a cellular level. By understanding the changes that occur in cells and tissue during disease states, researchers can develop new treatments to better target these diseases and improve patient outcomes.

In the case of immune system disorders, pathophysiology helps us better understand why certain individuals are more susceptible to certain diseases or why some treatments are more effective for certain individuals. For example, understanding the mechanisms behind immune system disorders can help researchers develop drugs that target specific pathways and prevent disease progression. In addition, pathophysiology can help us understand why certain treatments may not be as effective in some people, helping to inform better decisions on how to treat these diseases.

Pathophysiology can also help us better understand the role of environmental factors in disease. For example, exposure to certain pollutants or allergens may trigger an immune system response and lead to the development of allergies or asthma. By understanding how these environmental factors interact with the body, researchers can develop ways to prevent or mitigate their effects and improve patient outcomes.

Respiratory System

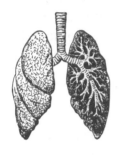

The respiratory system is a complex and crucial system in the human body, responsible for maintaining vital oxygen levels. Pathophysiology of the respiratory system can manifest itself in numerous ways, ranging from acute illnesses to chronic conditions. Acute illnesses such as bronchitis and pneumonia are caused by viruses or bacteria invading the lungs, causing inflammation which leads to difficulty breathing. Asthma is another common respiratory condition, where the airways become inflamed and narrowed, resulting in breathing difficulties. Chronic obstructive pulmonary disease (COPD) is largely caused by smoking and leads to irreversible deterioration of the lungs. In addition to a range of medications available for treating these conditions, lifestyle changes such as quitting smoking or reducing exposure to pollutants can help reduce symptoms.

Sleep apnea is another condition of the respiratory system, where breathing is interrupted during sleep. This can lead to snoring, excessive daytime sleepiness, and difficulty concentrating. Treatment for this condition usually involves lifestyle changes such as weight loss and avoiding alcohol or sleeping pills before bed. Additionally, surgery may be necessary in some cases, or the use of a continuous positive airway pressure (CPAP) machine to ensure constant air flow to the lungs.

Role Of Pathophysiology In Respiratory System Development

The body's pathophysiological processes play a crucial role in the development of respiratory diseases. When the lungs are healthy, they function optimally to deliver oxygen and remove carbon dioxide from the blood. However, when these functions become impaired due to disease or injury, pathological changes can occur which leads to respiratory illness. As certain conditions such as COPD progress and worsen, the damage to the lungs increases, leading to more severe breathing difficulties. The pathophysiology of COPD involves an inflammatory response within the lungs in which immune cells, cytokines, and oxidants are released, causing further destruction to the airways.

Pathophysiology is also involved in healthy respiratory development. For example, during fetal development, a process called lung maturation occurs, in which the lungs develop and prepare for breathing. This involves various changes such as surfactant production, increased blood flow, and formation of conducting airways. Understanding how these processes work can help diagnose conditions before they become severe.

The Steps Of Pathophysiology In Treating The Respiratory System

The treatment of respiratory illnesses involves a variety of steps, depending on the severity and type of condition. For mild cases, lifestyle changes such as avoiding triggers or using medications can help reduce symptoms. In more severe cases, surgery may be necessary to improve airway function or reduce inflammation in the lungs. Pathophysiological processes are also used in treatments, particularly for chronic conditions. For example, in COPD, medications such as bronchodilators can be used to reduce inflammation and open the airways, while anti-inflammatory drugs can help reduce or prevent further damage to the lungs.

In addition to medication and lifestyle changes, physical therapy can also be beneficial for respiratory illnesses. Physical therapists use specific exercises to strengthen the muscles of the chest and abdomen, which can help improve breathing. Pathophysiological processes are also involved in treatments for obstructive sleep apnea, such as the use of a CPAP machine to maintain consistent air flow to the lungs.

Overall, understanding pathophysiology is crucial for treating respiratory illnesses, both acute and chronic. With proper diagnosis and treatment plans, patients can reduce symptoms and improve their quality of life. By making lifestyle changes such as quitting smoking or reducing exposure to pollutants, people can help prevent respiratory illnesses from developing or worsening in the future. Understanding and treating pathophysiological processes is therefore an important part of maintaining healthy lungs.

Neurologic System

The nervous system consists of the central and peripheral nervous systems. The nervous system works together to coordinate information, control movement, regulate hormones, and much more. The brain is the main organ of the Central Nervous System (CNS) while the Peripheral Nervous System (PNS) includes all the nerves that extend from the CNS and reach out to the muscles and organs.

Neural Pathophysiology is the study of how diseases affect the nervous system, with a focus on vascular, mechanical, chemical and physiological changes. Examples of such diseases include stroke,

Alzheimer's disease, Lou Gehrig's disease (ALS), multiple sclerosis (MS) and Parkinson's Disease. Each disease affects specific parts of the nervous system, leading to a wide range of functional and physical deficits.

Neuroplasticity is the brain's ability to reorganize itself by forming new neural connections throughout life. This process can be used as a way to modify behaviour or adapt to neurological damage from diseases such as stroke, trauma or Alzheimer's disease. Neuroplasticity has been studied extensively and it is now believed that the brain can learn new skills, even if its structure or connections have been damaged.

The nervous system also contains a variety of sensory receptors, which help us process information from our environment. There are different categories of sensory receptors-thermoreceptors in the skin detect temperature changes, proprioceptive receptors sense body position and force, and photoreceptors detect light. Sensory receptors provide information to the brain that is used for decision-making, movement coordination or even emotion regulation.

Role Of Pathophysiology In Neurologic System Development

Pathophysiology plays an important role in the development and maintenance of the neurologic system. It helps to understand how changes in normal physiology impact brain function and associated structures. Pathophysiology also contributes to our understanding of how certain diseases, such as traumatic brain injury or dementia, affect the neurologic system.

By studying pathophysiology, we can identify and better understand the underlying processes that contribute to neurologic impairment. This can help us develop more effective treatments for these conditions, as well as preventative measures to reduce the risk of neurologic conditions in individuals.

Pathophysiology also provides insight into how certain medications and other treatments affect brain functioning. For example, some medications can have an effect on the autonomic nervous system and can cause the body to respond abnormally. Understanding how these medications interact with the neurologic system can help us better manage neurological conditions and improve patient outcomes.

Finally, pathophysiology enables us to study the effects of environmental factors on brain functioning. This includes studying how certain pollutants, such as heavy metals or toxins, impact brain functioning and behaviour. Understanding how these substances interact with the neurologic system can help us develop preventive strategies to reduce the risk of neurological disorders in individuals.

The Steps Of Pathophysiology In Treating The Neurologic System

The steps of pathophysiology in treating the neurologic system are as follows:

1. Diagnosis: This involves identifying the cause of neurological dysfunction. This requires an accurate diagnosis, which includes a detailed medical history and a physical examination.
2. Treatment: Once the underlying cause has been identified, appropriate treatment can be provided. This may include medications or therapies that address the underlying condition.
3. Follow-up: After treatment is complete, follow-up care is important to ensure that the neurologic symptoms have resolved. This may include additional testing or therapies, depending on the individual's case.
4. Prevention: Preventative strategies can also be implemented to reduce the likelihood of a recurrence of neurological dysfunction. These may include lifestyle changes, such as smoking cessation or healthy eating habits, and they may also include environmental modifications, such as improved air quality or water

contamination control.

Renal System

The renal system is made up of the two kidneys, which are located in the lower back. The primary function of the kidneys is to filter waste and excess water from our bodies, producing urine. Urine is composed of urea, electrolytes, creatinine, ammonia and other substances that can be toxic when present in excessive amounts.

The renal system also helps to keep our blood pressure in a healthy range. When there is an increase in the levels of sodium or potassium, the kidneys help regulate these concentrations so that they are kept within normal limits.

Pathophysiology of renal system refers to any abnormality or disorder of kidney function. These conditions can cause various symptoms such as edema, hypertension, proteinuria and electrolyte imbalance. Some of the more common causes of renal system pathophysiology include chronic kidney disease, diabetic nephropathy, glomerulonephritis and acute tubular necrosis.

These are just a few examples of conditions that can affect the renal system. Treatment for these conditions will usually involve medications such as diuretics, ACE inhibitors, or angiotensin receptor blockers. Other treatments, such as dialysis or kidney transplantation, may be needed in more severe cases.

Role Of Pathophysiology In Renal System Development

Pathophysiology plays an important role in the development of renal system disorders. The body's response to stress can affect the way that the kidneys respond to challenges, leading to changes in their function over time.

For example, when faced with long-term stress, such as chronic hypertension or diabetes, the renal system may not be properly equipped to handle the increased workload. As a result, the kidney's ability to properly filter out toxins and excess fluid can be compromised. This can lead to damage in the renal system such as glomerulosclerosis or nephropathy, both of which may require medical intervention for treatment.

In addition, certain medications and supplements that are taken over long periods of time can also affect the renal system. These include NSAIDs, antacids, and antibiotics, which can lead to a decrease in kidney function over time.

Therefore, it is important to be aware of any potential risks when taking medications or supplements that could potentially contribute to pathophysiology in the renal system. Doing so can help prevent unnecessary damage to the kidneys and help maintain their health. Making lifestyle changes that reduce stress and improve overall wellness can also help to protect the kidneys from pathophysiology.

By understanding how various conditions can affect the renal system, it is possible to take steps to reduce the risk of developing pathophysiological disorders in the future. With this knowledge, individuals can make informed decisions about treatments and medications that will help protect their kidneys and maintain a healthy renal system.

The Steps Of Pathophysiology In Treating The Renal System

In some cases, pathophysiology can be used to diagnose and treat disorders of the renal system. When a patient is suspected of having a problem with their kidneys, diagnostic tests such as urine tests, blood tests, and imaging studies are often ordered to determine the cause of the problem.

Once a diagnosis is made, treatment can then begin. Generally speaking, treatment for renal system disorders will involve medications, surgical interventions or lifestyle changes.

Medications such as diuretics and ACE inhibitors are commonly used to help reduce pressure on the kidneys and improve their ability to filter toxins from the body. In some cases, kidney transplantation may be necessary if a patient is no longer able to adequately filter wastes from their blood.

When it comes to lifestyle changes, making healthy choices such as following a balanced diet, exercising regularly and reducing stress can help improve kidney function and reduce the risk of developing renal system diseases. Even something as simple as drinking plenty of water each day can be beneficial for the kidneys.

Sensory System

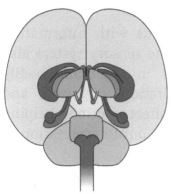

The human sensory system is a complex network of specialized cells and organs that allow us to experience and interpret the world around us. It involves mainly five senses: sight, hearing, smell, taste, and touch (also known as haptic). Each sense has specific receptors which detect different forms of energy—light, sound waves, odour molecules, flavours and pressure respectively.

The nervous system is the main organ of the sensory system, responsible for carrying out electrical impulses from the receptors to the brain and other parts of the body. This helps us to make sense of our environment and recognize different stimuli. For instance, when a person looks at an object, light waves are detected by special cells in their eyes, which then send electrical signals to the brain. The brain then interprets the input and the person is able to recognize the object.

The sensory system also works in reverse, sending messages from the brain through nerves to various organs of the body. This helps us control our movements and interpret sensations from our environment such as temperature, pain, or pleasure.

In addition to providing us with information about our environment, the sensory system also plays an important role in regulating bodily functions such as respiration, digestion, and reproduction. It can even affect emotions, helping us make decisions based on our interpretation of various stimuli.

Sensory disorders often occur when the sensory receptors become damaged or do not function correctly. This can result in a range of issues, such as hearing or vision loss, balance problems, and difficulty interpreting information. Treatment for sensory disorders can involve medications or devices that help to restore the function of the receptors and/or improve their performance.

Role Of Pathophysiology In Sensory System Disease Development

The pathophysiology of sensory system diseases can be described as the disturbance of normal bodily functions caused by damage to one or more of its components. Such disturbances may arise from a variety of factors, such as genetic defects, environmental exposures, infections, and other causes. In some instances, the cause is unknown.

One example of a sensory system disorder is deafness, which is caused by damage to the auditory nerve or inner ear. Hearing loss may be congenital (present at birth) or acquired during life and can range from mild to profound. Treatment of hearing loss depends upon its cause and degree of severity, but may include hearing aids, cochlear implants, assistive listening devices, speech therapy, and/or sign language.

The pathophysiology of visual system diseases may include damage to the retina, optic nerve, or visual pathway. Diseases such as glaucoma and macular degeneration can cause vision loss that may range from mild to severe. Treatment of these conditions typically involves medications, laser therapy, or surgery.

In addition to hearing and vision loss, the pathophysiology of other sensory system diseases includes taste disturbances (taste aversions), smell impairment, and tactile dysfunction. Treatment for these conditions may involve medications, lifestyle changes, or therapies such as aromatherapy in the case of smell impairment.

Sensory System Pathophysiology

The senses, such as sight, hearing, and touch, are controlled by the nervous system. When these systems fail to properly function due to diseases or malfunctioning of organs involved in the sensory process, it is called a pathology of the sensory system.

Many disorders of the sensory system can cause severe disability due to a lack of awareness and understanding of one's environment. These disorders can include hearing loss, deafness, vision impairment or blindness, sensory processing disorder (SPD), and dysfunctions in the sense of taste and smell.

Hearing loss is among the most common sensory system disorders, affecting up to 15% of people worldwide. It can be caused by environmental factors such as excessive noise, genetic factors, or aging. People with hearing loss may experience difficulty understanding conversations, tinnitus (a ringing in the ear), or balance issues.

Vision impairment is also a common sensory system disorder that can be caused by numerous conditions including glaucoma, macular degeneration, cataracts and retinal detachment. This condition can cause decreased vision, blindness, and even colour vision issues.

Sensory processing disorder (SPD) is an umbrella term for conditions in which the brain has difficulty processing information from the senses. Individuals with SPD may struggle with tactile sensitivity or seeking sensory input, have difficulties concentrating or focusing, or experience over-responsiveness to sounds and smells.

The sense of taste and smell can also be affected by pathophysiology. Taste is controlled by the gustatory cells in the tongue that interact with chemicals in foods to send signals to the brain. A disorder known as ageusia affects one's ability to taste, while anosmia, or an inability to smell can be caused by certain illnesses or head trauma.

Pathophysiology of the sensory system can cause serious disability if left untreated. If you or someone you know is struggling with a sensory disorder, it is important to contact your healthcare provider for treatment and support. Early identification and treatment may prevent further complications from arising.

Steps Of Sensory System Pathophysiology

The pathophysiology of the sensory system can be broken down into several distinct steps. Firstly, damage or alteration to the receptors in the peripheral nervous system will cause a decrease in sensation. Secondly, information from the receptors is transmitted along nerve pathways to processing centres where it is further processed and then finally sent on to higher cortical areas for interpretation. Thirdly, changes in neural pathways due to pathology can affect the accuracy of information sent along them. Finally, any disruption of higher cortical areas or changes in cognitive function can lead to misinterpretation or misperception of sensory input.

In addition, there are certain conditions which can cause a heightened level of sensitivity to sensory stimuli. For example, hyperacusis is an increase in sound sensitivity caused by an auditory abnormality, and hyperalgesia is an increase in sensitivity to pain caused by damage to the peripheral nervous system. Furthermore, certain medical conditions such as fibromyalgia can cause widespread sensory problems throughout the body.

It's important to note that the pathophysiology of the sensory system can manifest itself through a wide range of signs and symptoms which must be carefully considered in order to get an accurate diagnosis. Symptoms could range from decreased sensitivity to increased sensitivity and can affect any of the five senses; hearing, sight, smell, taste and touch. Other symptoms such as cognitive impairments may also manifest depending on the underlying cause of a sensory problem.

Ultimately, understanding how pathophysiology affects the sensory system is an important part of diagnosing and treating any medical condition which affects it. By taking a comprehensive approach to diagnosis, doctors can ensure the best possible outcomes for their patients.

Finally, it's worth noting that advances in neuroscience have allowed researchers to gain a greater understanding of how the brain processes sensory signals. This research has led to more effective treatments for many neurological and sensory disorders, as well as improved diagnosis and management of existing conditions. This is leading to a greater quality of life for those affected by sensory pathologies.

Reproductive System

The reproductive system allows us to reproduce and bring new life into the world. It is composed of several parts that all work together to make it possible for a baby to be born. The main organs of the reproductive system are the ovaries, uterus, fallopian tubes, and vagina in women; and the testes, epididymis, scrotum, and penis in men.

The ovaries are the female gonads which produce eggs or ova. The uterus is a muscular organ located inside the pelvis that houses a fertilized egg during pregnancy until it is ready for delivery through the vagina. The fallopian tubes connect the ovaries to the uterus and allow sperm to travel from outside of the body to meet the egg in the ovary. The vagina is a tube-like organ that serves as the passage for sperm to meet an egg and also as a delivery canal for giving birth.

The testes are male gonads which produce sperm. The epididymis is a small, coiled tube where immature sperm cells mature as they move towards the prostate gland. The scrotum is a loose pouch of skin that hangs below the penis and holds the testicles in place for proper temperature regulation. Finally, the penis is an organ responsible for sexual intercourse and delivering semen from the male body to fertilize an egg in a woman's reproductive system.

The reproductive system also consists of hormones that are essential for sexual activity and reproduction. These hormones are produced in the hypothalamus, pituitary gland, testes, and ovaries. The hormones produced control things such as puberty, fertility, and even mood.

In addition to these organs and hormones, the reproductive system also performs other important functions that contribute to the health of individuals in many ways. For example, the reproductive system provides immunity to help protect us from diseases and other illnesses. It also plays a role in maintaining psychological balance by providing a sense of self-identity and purpose for individuals.

Reproductive System Pathophysiology

Pathophysiology is the study of how diseases develop and progress. The reproductive system is prone to a variety of pathologies, such as infertility, ectopic pregnancy, ovarian cysts, endometriosis, and sexually transmitted infections (STIs).

Infertility can occur due to structural or functional problems with the ovaries, uterus, fallopian tubes, or sperm production. If the egg is unable to be fertilized due to an anatomical abnormality or a lack of motility in the sperm, this can result in infertility.

Ectopic pregnancy is when a fertilized egg implants outside of the uterus, such as in the fallopian tube. This condition can cause severe pain and must be treated immediately.

Ovarian cysts are fluid-filled sacs that can form on the ovaries and may cause pelvic pain or abnormal bleeding. These cysts can be benign or malignant, so it is important to discuss any symptoms with your healthcare provider.

Endometriosis occurs when the tissue that lines the uterus (endometrium) grows outside of the uterus. This can cause abdominal pain, cramping, and other symptoms depending on where the tissue is growing.

STIs can be spread through sexual contact and can include bacterial or viral infections. Common STIs include gonorrhoea, chlamydia, HIV/AIDS, genital herpes, hepatitis B, syphilis, and trichomoniasis. Symptoms vary depending on the infection and can include pain, itching, unusual discharge, or sores. It is important to be tested for STIs if you have had unprotected sex or are experiencing any symptoms.

Pathophysiology of the reproductive system involves understanding how diseases of this system develop and progress in order to provide effective diagnosis and treatment. Taking preventive measures such as practicing safe sex or getting regular screenings can help reduce the risk of diseases in the reproductive system.

Additionally, understanding how to recognize symptoms and when to seek medical attention is important for maintaining reproductive health. Early detection of any problems can provide better treatment options and help reduce long-term complications. Working with a healthcare specialist who specializes in reproductive health issues can help ensure that your reproductive health is maintained.

Role Of Pathophysiology In Reproductive System Disease Development

Pathophysiology is an important concept in understanding the development of diseases in the reproductive system. It involves the study of changes in normal physiological processes that lead to disease or altered health states. Pathological changes can involve the structure and/or function of organs, tissues, cells, and molecules.

When studying reproductive system diseases, pathophysiological principles can be used to understand the underlying causes of disease. This includes understanding changes in hormones, receptors, enzymes, proteins, and other molecules that are involved in the reproductive system. For example, an imbalance between estrogen and progesterone is commonly associated with infertility or dysfunctional uterine bleeding. Understanding how these hormones interact can help diagnose and manage reproductive system diseases.

Pathophysiology also helps explain the mechanisms by which diseases develop in the reproductive system. It can provide insight into how environmental and lifestyle factors, such as diet, exposure to toxins, or exercise, may contribute to an individual's risk of developing a particular condition. For example, research has shown that poor nutrition can increase an individual's risk for endometriosis and infertility.

Pathophysiology can also be used to assess and monitor treatment efficacy. By understanding how changes in hormones, receptors, enzymes, proteins, and other molecules affect reproductive system disease progression or remission, physicians can adjust therapies to ensure optimal results.

Steps Of Reproductive System Pathophysiology

Reproductive system pathophysiology is the study of the abnormal functioning of the reproductive organs. It includes a variety of diseases, syndromes and conditions that affect reproductive organ function. The most common problems include infertility, endometriosis, fibroids, polycystic ovarian syndrome (PCOS), and pelvic inflammatory disease (PID).

The first step in diagnosing reproductive system pathophysiology is to get an accurate medical history and physical examination. During the medical history, doctors will ask questions about your health, family history, sexual lifestyle, and any current symptoms you may be experiencing. A physical exam will also help identify any underlying issues that could be responsible for your symptoms.

The second step in diagnosing reproductive system pathophysiology is to have blood tests, imaging tests, and other laboratory tests performed. Blood tests help to detect hormone levels and abnormalities in the body's chemistry that could be responsible for infertility or any other symptoms you are experiencing. Imaging tests such as ultrasounds can also provide important information about your reproductive organs and any underlying issues that could be causing your symptoms.

The third step in diagnosing reproductive system pathophysiology is to have a laparoscopy or hysteroscopy performed. These procedures allow the doctor to take a look inside the pelvis and uterus using specialized cameras and instruments. During these procedures, doctors can identify any anatomical problems that could be contributing to your fertility problems or other symptoms.

The fourth step in diagnosing reproductive system pathophysiology is to have a hysterosalpingogram (HSG) test performed. This test uses contrast dye injected into the uterus and fallopian tubes which can highlight any blockages or abnormalities that could be hindering the ability for egg fertilization.

Finally, the fifth step in diagnosing reproductive system pathophysiology is to have a laparotomy performed. This procedure involves making an incision through the abdomen and pelvic region to allow further examination of the internal organs. Laparotomies are usually only recommended if other non-invasive methods do not yield useful results or if there are more serious underlying health concerns at play that need to be addressed.

By following these five steps, doctors can accurately diagnose any reproductive system pathophysiology and develop a treatment plan that is appropriate for the patient's individual needs. Treatment plans may include medications, lifestyle changes, or surgical interventions depending on the underlying cause of the condition. It is important to remember that with early diagnosis and proper care, many reproductive system pathophysiology issues can be effectively managed.

CHAPTER 4: AUTOIMMUNE
DISEASES

Autoimmune diseases are a group of disorders in which the patient's own immune system attacks healthy cells and tissues, instead of targeting foreign substances such as bacteria or viruses. Examples of common autoimmune diseases include lupus, type 1 diabetes, rheumatoid arthritis, multiple sclerosis, and Crohn's disease. Autoimmune diseases can affect virtually any part of the body, including the skin, joints, organs, and muscles. Depending on the type of autoimmune disease, symptoms can range from mild to severe and can include fatigue, joint pain or swelling, fever, rash or lesions on the skin, difficulty breathing or swallowing, and organ malfunction. Treatment for autoimmune diseases typically involves medications to suppress the overactive immune system with corticosteroids and non-steroidal anti-inflammatory drugs, or immunosuppressants to limit the immune system's activity. In some cases, surgery may be required to remove damaged organs.

Lupus

Lupus is an autoimmune condition which causes the body to create antibodies that attack healthy cells, leading to symptoms such as joint pain, fatigue and a rash on the cheeks and nose. It can have serious consequences if left untreated, including damage to the heart, lungs and kidneys. Treatment for lupus usually involves medications such as steroids or immunosuppressive drugs. Surgery may also be required in some cases. Early diagnosis and aggressive treatment are essential to reducing the severity of lupus symptoms and preventing more serious complications.

Lupus Pathophysiology

The exact pathophysiology of lupus is still unknown, however, it is believed that genetic and environmental factors may play a role. Several genes have been linked to the development of lupus, including ones found in the human leukocyte antigen (HLA) system. Environmental triggers such as UV light exposure, certain medications and infections may also cause lupus to flare up.

Once the immune system has been triggered, it begins attacking healthy cells and tissues, resulting in inflammation throughout the body. The inflammation can cause damage to organs and tissues, leading to further symptoms such as joint pain, fatigue and the classic 'butterfly rash' on the face. In some cases, lupus can cause serious complications such as kidney failure, heart attack and stroke.

Type 1 Diabetes

Type 1 diabetes is an autoimmune disease that

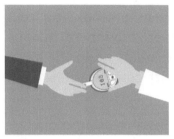

affects millions of people around the world. The body's immune system mistakenly attacks and destroys the cells in the pancreas that produce insulin, a hormone essential for controlling blood sugar levels. Without insulin, glucose builds up in the blood and can cause serious health complications in individuals with type 1 diabetes.

In order to manage the condition, individuals with type 1 diabetes must regularly monitor their blood sugar levels and administer insulin injections to regulate their glucose levels. Additionally, a balanced diet and regular physical activity are essential for those living with this chronic condition.

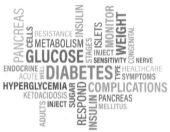

Type 1 Diabetes Pathophysiology

The exact cause of type 1 diabetes is still unclear, however, it is believed to be related to genetics and environmental factors. The body's immune system mistakenly attacks and destroys the cells in the pancreas that produce insulin. These toxins are known as autoantibodies and can be detected in the blood of individuals with type 1 diabetes.

The destruction of the insulin-producing cells causes a decrease in the production of insulin. When this occurs, glucose builds up in the blood and can lead to serious health complications if left unchecked.

Treatment for type 1 diabetes typically involves lifestyle changes such as following a balanced diet and regular physical activity, as well as monitoring and administering insulin injections on a regular basis. Additionally, monitoring of blood sugar levels is essential to ensure that glucose does not reach dangerously high levels.

By making lifestyle changes and following the doctor's advice, individuals with type 1 diabetes can live a healthy and active life. With careful management, serious health complications caused by this condition can be avoided.

Rheumatoid Arthritis Diagnosis

Diagnosing rheumatoid arthritis is based on a combination of clinical presentation, laboratory tests, and imaging studies. A physical examination will assess joint function, swelling, tenderness, and range of motion. Blood tests can detect inflammation markers such as erythrocyte sedimentation rate (ESR) or C-reactive protein (CRP). Imaging studies such as X-rays or magnetic resonance imaging (MRI) can reveal joint damage.

Rheumatoid arthritis is a chronic disease

and there is no cure; however, early diagnosis and aggressive treatment can help slow the progression of the disease and improve the patient's quality of life. A team approach involving rheumatologists, primary care physicians, physical therapists, and mental health practitioners is important for the successful management of patients with RA.

The key takeaway is that rheumatoid arthritis diagnosis involves a combination of clinical evaluation, laboratory tests, and imaging studies. Early diagnosis and aggressive treatment can help slow disease progression and improve quality of life. A team approach involving multiple specialists can provide better care for patients with RA.

Rheumatoid Arthritis Pathophysiology

Rheumatoid arthritis (RA) is an autoimmune disorder characterized by inflammation of the synovial membrane and joints. The cause of RA is not yet known; however, genetic factors are believed to play a role in its development.

The pathogenesis involves the immune system attacking the joint structures resulting in inflammation and cartilage damage. The inflammation of the synovial membrane leads to an increased production of pro-inflammatory cytokines which further damages the cartilage and bones. This ultimately leads to joint destruction and deformity, pain, stiffness, and a decrease in physical activity.

RA is associated with other comorbidities such as cardiovascular disease, osteoporosis, depression, anxiety, and fatigue. Treatment for rheumatoid arthritis includes medications to help reduce inflammation and pain, as well as physical therapy, lifestyle changes, and surgery. With proper treatment, the symptoms of RA can be managed and patients can live a relatively normal life.

The key takeaway is that rheumatoid arthritis is an autoimmune disease with unknown causes but likely genetic contributions. It is associated with joint destruction and pain, stiffness, as well as other comorbidities. Treatment for RA includes medications, physical therapy, lifestyle changes, and surgery to manage symptoms and improve quality of life.

Multiple Sclerosis

Multiple sclerosis (MS) is an immune-mediated disease of the central nervous system (CNS). In MS, the immune system attacks and destroys myelin, a type of protective sheath that surrounds nerve cells. The destruction of this protective layer inhibits communication between the brain and other parts of the body, leading to muscle weakness, impaired coordination, vision problems, fatigue and other symptoms.

MS is a progressive disease, meaning that it can worsen over time. The exact cause of MS is still unknown, however, environmental factors and genetics are both thought to play a role in its development. Risk factors for developing MS include being female, having family members with the disease, living in certain geographic regions, smoking and viral infections.

Multiple Sclerosis Pathophysiology

In MS, the body's own immune system mistakenly attacks the myelin sheath that surrounds nerve cells, causing inflammation and scarring. This damage disrupts communication between the brain and other parts of the body. As a result, individuals with MS experience muscle weakness, impaired coordination, vision problems, fatigue and other symptoms related to disruption in neural pathways.

The exact pathway by which the body's immune system begins to attack myelin is still not fully understood. In some cases, an environmental trigger such as a virus can set off the immune system and initiate the attack on myelin. However, other cases of MS do not appear to be triggered by any known environmental factor.

In addition to attacking myelin, the body's immune system may also attack neurons in certain areas of the brain. This can lead to additional neurological symptoms, such as difficulty speaking or thinking clearly.

MS is a complex condition and the pathophysiology of the disease is still not fully understood. Research into this area continues in an effort to further understand and improve treatments for MS.

Crohn's Disease Pathophysiology

Crohn's disease is a chronic, or long-term, inflammatory condition that affects the lining of the digestive tract. It is one of two types of Inflammatory Bowel Disease (IBD) and most commonly develops in those aged 16 to 25 years old.

The pathophysiology behind Crohn's disease is complex and not fully understood. It is believed that it may be caused by a combination of genetic, environmental and immunological factors. In susceptible individuals, inflammation in the digestive tract occurs when their immune system mistakenly attacks healthy tissue as if it were an invader or virus. This triggers an inflammatory response and can lead to pain, cramping, diarrhoea, weight loss and anaemia.

Crohn's disease can affect any part of the digestive tract, from the mouth to the anus. The inflammation is often patchy and may spread deep into the layers of your bowel wall. This can cause scarring, fistulas (abnormal connections between organs) or obstruction (blockage in your intestine).

Inflammation caused by Crohn's disease can also cause other serious health issues, such as arthritis, skin rashes, eye problems or liver and bile duct inflammation. It is important to receive early diagnosis and treatment to help prevent these complications.

Treating Crohn's disease often involves medications, such as anti-inflammatory drugs or immunosuppressants (which reduce the body's immune response). Surgery may also be needed in some cases to remove severely damaged areas of the intestine. Dietary changes, such as reducing dairy products or avoiding certain foods, can also help reduce symptoms.

Advanced Understanding Of Crohn's Disease Pathophysiology

While the pathophysiology of Crohn's disease remains incompletely understood, recent advancements in medical research suggest the role of gut microbiota in its development. The human gut harbors a complex ecosystem of microbes, which contribute to maintaining gut health. However, an imbalance in this microbiota, known as dysbiosis, has been linked to Crohn's disease.

People with Crohn's often show a reduction in gut microbial diversity, with an increase in harmful bacteria and a decrease in beneficial ones. This dysbiosis may result in increased permeability of the gut lining, allowing bacteria and toxins to cross the intestinal barrier and trigger the immune system, thus exacerbating the inflammatory response.

Research is presently focused on understanding how to restore the balance of gut microbiota to treat or manage Crohn's disease. Probiotics, prebiotics, fecal microbiota transplant (FMT), and dietary changes are being studied for their potential in reducing inflammation and promoting gut health in those with Crohn's.

Further research is needed to fully understand this complex disease and develop more effective treatments. Until then, managing Crohn's disease involves reducing symptoms, maintaining nutritional status, and improving the quality of life for patients.

CHAPTER 5 : INFECTIOUS DISEASES

Infectious diseases are caused by microorganisms like bacteria, viruses, fungi, and parasites that can enter the body and cause severe damage. Common infectious diseases include the flu, chickenpox, HIV/AIDS, malaria, and measles. Symptoms of infectious diseases vary depending on the type of microorganism causing the infection; however, they can commonly include fever, coughing, headaches, vomiting or diarrhoea, joint pain or stiffness, rash or lesions on the skin, and difficulty breathing. Treatment for infectious diseases typically involves antibiotics or antiviral drugs to kill the microorganism or other medications for symptom relief. Vaccinations are also available to protect against certain types of infectious diseases.

Flu Disease

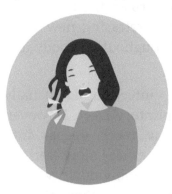

The flu is an acute, contagious respiratory infection caused by influenza viruses. It can affect people of all ages and can be dangerous for young children, pregnant women, the elderly, and those with weakened immune systems. Symptoms include fever, cough, sore throat, runny nose, muscle aches and fatigue.

Complications from the flu can range from mild to severe, such as bronchitis, pneumonia and even death. People with chronic health conditions such as asthma or heart disease are at higher risk of developing more serious complications.

Prevention of the flu includes getting an annual flu vaccine, washing hands often and avoiding close contact with people who are sick. Treatment for the flu is generally supportive and may include over-the-counter medications to reduce fever and pain, as well as drinking plenty of fluids. Antiviral drugs may be prescribed in some cases to help shorten the duration of symptoms.

Flu Pathophysiology

The pathophysiology of the flu begins when influenza virus particles attach to the cells lining the respiratory tract. The viruses then enter the cell and begin to replicate, releasing new virus particles which spread throughout the body and cause infection.

In healthy individuals, infection is usually limited to the upper respiratory tract. However, in some cases, virus may reach deeper into the respiratory tract and cause more serious symptoms. Additionally, in individuals with a weakened immune system or other chronic health conditions, the virus can spread to other parts of the body causing complications such as pneumonia or inflammation of the heart muscle (myocarditis).

Immune system responses to influenza infection include the production of antibodies which help destroy viruses and limit their spread throughout the body. In some cases, the immune response is inadequate and can lead to more severe symptoms or complications. Additionally, in people with weakened immune systems, the virus may replicate unchecked which can cause a more serious infection.

Understanding the pathophysiology of flu is essential for prevention and treatment of this condition. Vaccination against influenza viruses is important to reduce the risk of infection, while medications can help reduce the severity of symptoms and duration of illness. Additionally, good hygiene practices such as washing hands often and avoiding contact with those who are sick can help prevent the spread of the flu virus.

Chickenpox

Chickenpox is a highly contagious infection caused by the varicella-zoster virus. It is characterized by a red, itchy rash, which typically appears on the face, chest and back. The rash usually develops into small fluid-filled blisters that eventually break open and crust over. Other common symptoms of chickenpox include fever, headache, sore throat, chills and fatigue.

While chickenpox used to be a common childhood illness in the United States, it is now less common due to widespread vaccination. The vaccine is highly effective at preventing chickenpox, although it does not guarantee complete protection from the virus. Those who have been vaccinated can still develop a milder form of the disease with fewer symptoms.

Chickenpox is spread through contact with an infected person or their saliva. It can also be transmitted through airborne droplets when an infected person sneezes or coughs. Once a person has been infected, it usually takes two to three weeks for the symptoms to appear.

Most cases of chickenpox clear up within a few weeks without any long-term effects. However, some people may develop complications such as pneumonia and encephalitis. Those who have weakened immune systems or existing health conditions are at a higher risk of developing complications from the virus.

Chickenpox Pathophysiology

The pathophysiology of chickenpox involves the varicella-zoster virus entering the body and replicating in the lymph nodes. The virus then spreads through the bloodstream to other parts of the body, causing a rash to develop two to three weeks after the initial infection.

Once inside a cell, the virus contains genetic material that instructs it to make proteins known as "antigens". These antigens are responsible for triggering the body's immune response, causing inflammation and developing a rash. The body then produces antibodies to fight off the virus, which allows the infection to eventually clear up.

While most people recover from chickenpox without complications, some may develop post-viral neurological symptoms such as shingles (a virus related to chickenpox). Those who have contracted an extreme form of the virus may also be at risk for developing chronic skin conditions or breathing difficulties.

Treatment for chickenpox typically involves relieving symptoms and preventing further spread of the infection. A vaccine is available that can help prevent the disease, although it does not provide complete protection against the virus. Treatment may also involve antiviral medications or other treatments to reduce itching and inflammation. Those at a higher risk of developing complications should be monitored closely during treatment.

HIV/AIDS

HIV/AIDs is an acronym for Human Immunodeficiency Virus / Acquired Immune Deficiency Syndrome. It is a virus that can lead to a number of serious health complications, including

AIDS. HIV/AIDS is spread through contact with the body fluids of an infected person, such as semen or blood. It can also be transmitted from mother to child during childbirth or breastfeeding.

HIV is a virus that infects and damages the immune system, making it difficult for the body to fight off infection and disease. AIDS is the most advanced stage of HIV infection when someone has had either very low CD4 T-cell counts (less than 200) for more than three months or any opportunistic infections like cancer or tuberculosis.

Once someone has HIV, it is not curable but can be treated with antiretroviral therapy (ART). ART is a combination of drugs that help suppress the virus and keep it from reproducing. Treatment can slow down the progression of the disease and allow people with HIV to lead longer and healthier lives.

It's important to know the signs and symptoms of HIV/AIDS so that you can get tested and treated as soon as possible. Common symptoms of HIV/AIDS include fever, night sweats, weight loss, fatigue, swollen lymph nodes, and thrush (a yeast infection in the mouth).

HIV/AIDS And Pathophysiology

Pathophysiology refers to the study of changes in body function that occur as a result of disease or injury. In HIV/AIDS, pathophysiological changes occur throughout the body's vital organs and systems. Pathophysiologic changes include damage to the immune system, disruption of cell metabolism, inflammation, and production of toxic molecules.

The immune system is particularly affected by HIV/AIDS, as it leads to progressive depletion of CD4+ T-cells and macrophages, which play a vital role in defending the body from infection and disease. This can lead to an increased risk of opportunistic infections such as tuberculosis, (PCP) and cryptococcal meningitis.

HIV/AIDS can also cause damage to the nervous system, leading to peripheral neuropathy, cognitive decline, and HIV-associated dementia. Damage to the gastrointestinal system can result in diarrhoea, malabsorption syndrome, and other digestive issues. In addition, HIV/AIDS may cause kidney dysfunction and failure as well as organ failure.

Finally, HIV/AIDS can cause a range of other medical problems such as anaemia, osteoporosis, and skin disorders. In some cases, individuals living with HIV/AIDS may also experience psychological issues such as depression and anxiety.

These pathophysiological changes have a profound impact on individuals living with HIV/AIDS, which can cause serious physical and mental health consequences. It is important to recognize the potential for these changes in order to provide effective treatment and support.

Malaria

Malaria is a life-threatening parasitic infection caused by Plasmodium parasites. These parasites are spread through the bite of an infected female Anopheles mosquito and can cause symptoms such as fever, chills, headaches, nausea, vomiting, and muscle pain. In some cases, malaria can lead to severe complications such as brain damage or death. Treatment for malaria includes antimalarial medications and prompt medical care. It is important to note that there is no vaccine available for malaria, so prevention of infection primarily involves avoiding mosquito bites.

Malaria can be classified into four main types: falciparum, vivax, ovale, and malariae. Plasmodium falciparum is the most severe form of malaria and is responsible for the majority of malaria-related deaths worldwide. Plasmodium vivax is generally considered to be less serious than falciparum, but can still cause significant illness. It has been estimated that up to 300 million people are at risk of acquiring malaria every year, with approximately 90% of cases occurring in sub-Saharan Africa.

Malaria is a preventable and curable disease, yet it continues to be one of the world's major public health problems. In order to reduce the burden of malaria, effective control strategies must be implemented on a global level. These include vector control measures such as insecticide-treated bed nets, the use of antimalarial drugs for prevention and treatment of infection, and improved access to diagnosis and treatment. In addition, community education on measures that can be taken to reduce the risk of malaria infection will help to further decrease the burden of this deadly disease.

How Is Malaria Diagnosed?

Malaria is typically diagnosed through a blood test called the malaria rapid diagnostic test (mRDT). This test detects the presence of malaria parasites in a patient's bloodstream. If the mRDT is positive, additional tests may be performed to confirm the diagnosis and determine which type of malaria is present. Treatment for malaria typically involves antimalarial medications, such as chloroquine or artemisinin-based combination therapies (ACTs). It is important to note that antimalarial medications are only effective if taken as prescribed and monitored by a healthcare professional.

In some cases, malaria can also be diagnosed through other methods such as microscopy or PCR (polymerase chain reaction). Microscopy involves examining the patient's blood under a microscope to look for the presence of malaria parasites. PCR is a laboratory test that uses genetic material from the parasites to identify the species and determine which type of malaria is present.

Malaria Pathophysiology

The pathophysiology of malaria is complex and involves multiple organs and systems. The Plasmodium parasite has a complex life cycle which includes both the mosquito vector and the human host. After the infected mosquito bites a person, it injects Plasmodium sporozoites into their skin. These sporozoites then travel through the bloodstream to the liver where they begin to replicate. The liver is the major site of growth for Plasmodium and, as the infection progresses, it induces an inflammatory response which can lead to fever, chills, headaches, nausea, vomiting and muscle pain.

The parasite then moves out of the liver cells and into the red blood cells where it begins to multiply rapidly. This rapid replication of the parasite causes red blood cells to burst, resulting in anaemia and other symptoms. In severe cases, the infection can cause damage to other organs such as the brain or lungs.

Measles

Measles is a highly infectious disease caused by the measles virus. It is spread through contact with infected droplets, which are released into the air when an infected person coughs or sneezes. Symptoms usually appear seven to fourteen days after being exposed to the virus and can range from mild to severe. Common symptoms include fever, sore throat, cough, red eyes, and a telltale rash. In some cases, it can cause serious complications like pneumonia and encephalitis. Vaccination is the best way to prevent measles infections.

Measles Pathophysiology

The pathophysiology of measles begins when the virus is inhaled through respiratory droplets. Once inside the body, it attaches to and infects cells in the upper respiratory tract. It then multiplies and travels to regional lymph nodes, where it spreads further throughout the body. In severe cases, measles can spread to organs like the brain and intestine, leading to various complications.

The body's immune system responds to the infection by producing antibodies that fight against the virus. These antibodies help clear the virus from the body, but they can take up to two weeks to become effective. During this time, symptoms of measles can appear and worsen, including high fever, chills, mucous discharge from the eyes and nose and a red, blotchy rash. In rare cases, measles can cause inflammation of the brain or other organs, which can lead to serious complications like encephalitis.

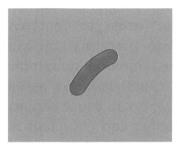

Tuberculosis

Tuberculosis, or TB, is an infectious disease caused by Mycobacterium tuberculosis. It is spread through inhaling tiny drops of infected saliva from a person with active TB. Common symptoms include fever, fatigue, night sweats, weight loss, and chest pain. Treatment typically involves antibiotics for several months to prevent the spread of the bacteria. Additionally, it is important to take steps to limit the spread of TB, such as avoiding contact with anyone who has active infection and practicing good hygiene.

Diagnosis And Testing For Tuberculosis

The diagnosis of TB is made through a combination of medical history, physical examination, chest x-rays, laboratory tests, and sputum culture. A chest x-ray can help detect any abnormalities in the lungs caused by the infection. Blood tests may also be used to look for antibodies to the bacteria that cause TB. Sputum cultures are used to identify the presence of TB bacteria in saliva and sputum samples.

Tuberculosis Pathophysiology

The mycobacterium tuberculosis is a type of bacteria that lives in the environment and usually causes infection when a person inhales tiny drops of saliva from an infected person. Once inside the body, the bacteria can grow in any part of the respiratory system. The infection can cause inflammation and tissue damage in the lungs and surrounding tissues, leading to symptoms such as fever, fatigue, night sweats, weight loss, and chest pain.

TB can spread through contact with fluids from an infected person's respiratory system. It is important to practice good hygiene, such as washing hands regularly and avoiding contact with anyone who has a known active infection of TB. Additionally, it is important to get tested for TB if you have been exposed to someone with the infection.

Lyme Disease

Lyme disease is a bacterial infection caused by Borrelia burgdorferi, a species of spirochete bacteria that are transmitted through the bite of an infected black-legged tick. These ticks are found in many wooded and grassy areas across North America. Lyme disease can be difficult to diagnose because its symptoms vary from person to person, and many of them are similar to the symptoms of other diseases.

The most common symptom of Lyme disease is a circular rash that appears at the site of the tick bite. This rash may be accompanied by flu-like symptoms such as fever, fatigue, chills, muscle aches, and joint pain. If not treated early on, the infection can spread to other parts of the body, causing neurological and cardiac symptoms.

Left untreated, Lyme disease can lead to serious complications such as arthritis, cognitive difficulties, and facial palsy. It's important to seek medical attention right away if you think you might have been exposed to Lyme disease—the earlier it is diagnosed and treated, the better the outcome for the patient.

Lyme Disease Pathophysiology

The pathophysiology of Lyme disease begins with a bite from an infected black-legged tick, which transmits the Borrelia burgdorferi spirochete bacteria into the body. Once in the body, the bacteria can then spread to other parts of the body via the circulatory system. As it spreads, it produces toxins that create an inflammatory response, causing the characteristic rash as well as other symptoms such as fever, fatigue, and joint pain.

The bacteria can also cause damage to the heart, joints, and nervous system if left untreated. It is believed that this is caused by an autoimmune reaction triggered by the presence of Borrelia burgdorferi in the body. If left untreated for too long, the damage done by the bacteria can be irreversible.

Fortunately, Lyme disease is treatable if caught early enough. Treatment typically consists of antibiotics, which help to kill off the bacteria and reduce inflammation. If left untreated or treated too late, however, it can lead to serious complications that can cause lasting damage. For this reason, it's important to seek medical attention as soon as you suspect that you may have been exposed to Lyme disease. Early diagnosis and treatment are key to ensuring a successful outcome.

Ebola

Ebola is a virus that causes an infectious disease in humans and other primates. It is one of two members of the family Filoviridae, along with Marburg virus. Ebola's symptoms can be severe and often include fever, intense weakness, muscle pain, headache and sore throat followed by vomiting, diarrhoea, rash, impaired kidney and liver function, and in some cases, both internal and external bleeding. The average case fatality rate is around 50%, making it one of the world's most virulent diseases.

There is currently no approved treatment or vaccine for Ebola, despite ongoing research efforts. Treatment consists of providing supportive care such as fluids and electrolytes to prevent dehydration and rehydrate patients; treating other infections if they occur; and optimizing oxygen levels and blood pressure. Patients can become carriers of the virus when they are not cured of the disease, which makes prevention strategies such as contact tracing crucial to controlling outbreaks. Vaccines have been developed but are still in the clinical trial phase.

Ebola is believed to originate in fruit bats, however, it has been passed on to humans and other primates through contact with infected animals or people. Outbreaks occur mostly in remote villages of Central and West Africa, near tropical rainforests due to their close proximity to wildlife reservoirs. However, there have been cases reported in the United States, Italy, Spain and the Philippines. The risk of an outbreak is highest among people who come into contact with infected animals or individuals, such as healthcare workers and family members.

Once a person is infected with the virus, it can spread rapidly through contact with body fluids such as saliva, blood or vomit. In some cases, even touching contaminated objects such as clothing can lead to infection. Therefore, it is important to practice good hygiene and wear protective gear when caring for a patient.

Ebola Pathophysiology

Ebola is a negative-strand RNA virus of the family Filoviridae. It can cause severe and often fatal diseases in humans and other primates. The virus has an incubation period of 2 to 21 days before symptoms begin to appear.

Once inside the body, Ebola replicates rapidly within cells and interferes with the cells' normal functioning. It can cause disruption of the immune system, damage to blood vessels, and inflammation of organs such as the liver and kidneys. This leads to a range of symptoms including fever, fatigue, headache, nausea and vomiting, rash, joint and muscle pain, bleeding from multiple sites in the body (hemorrhaging), organ failure and death.

Ebola is spread through direct contact with body fluids from an infected person or animal. It can also be spread indirectly when people come into contact with objects that have been contaminated with the virus (such as clothing, bedding, needles, and medical equipment).

The mortality rate of Ebola outbreaks varies from 25% to 90%, depending on the strain of virus and access to medical care. However, early detection and supportive treatment can help reduce the mortality rate significantly. Treatment includes providing fluids and electrolytes to prevent dehydration, treating other infections if they occur, optimizing oxygen levels and blood pressure, and providing supportive care such as pain relief. There is currently no approved vaccine or specific treatment for Ebola, although research efforts are ongoing. The best way to prevent infection is to practice good hygiene, wear protective gear when caring for a patient, and avoid contact with infected animals or people.

It is important that healthcare professionals are trained in the diagnosis and treatment of Ebola and other similar diseases, as well as how to properly handle and dispose of infectious materials. In addition, public health measures such as contact tracing and education are essential in preventing the spread of this deadly virus. With the right knowledge and resources, we can all help to protect ourselves and others from Ebola and its devastating effects.

CHAPTER 6: DIGESTIVE DISEASES

Digestive diseases occur when there is abnormal functioning of the digestive organs such as the stomach, intestines, and liver. Common examples of digestive diseases are irritable bowel syndrome, ulcerative colitis, and gastroesophageal reflux disease. Symptoms of digestive diseases can include abdominal pain or discomfort, bloating or gas, diarrhoea or constipation, nausea and vomiting, heartburn and acid reflux, weight loss or gain, and fatigue. Treatment for digestive diseases can involve medications, lifestyle changes, or surgery depending on the severity of the condition.

Irritable Bowel Syndrome

Irritable bowel syndrome (IBS) is one of the most common chronic gastrointestinal disorders in adults, affecting up to 10-15% of the population. IBS is a functional disorder that affects how the muscles of the large intestine work, leading to abdominal pain and discomfort, bloating, and changes in bowel habits. Symptoms vary from person to person and can fluctuate over time.

The exact cause of IBS is unknown but it is believed to be related to a combination of factors, including genetics, the environment, the immune system, diet, and stress. People with IBS often have an imbalance in their gut bacteria (microbiome) that can lead to increased sensitivity in the digestive tract and changes in the way food moves through the digestive system.

IBS is diagnosed based on the symptoms experienced by an individual, as there is no specific test that can be used to diagnose IBS. Treatment of IBS is tailored to the individual and may include dietary changes, stress management, regular exercise, medication, or psychotherapy. It is important for people with IBS to find a doctor they can trust and develop a good working relationship with in order to best manage their symptoms.

IBS is a chronic condition, but some steps can be taken to reduce or manage the symptoms and improve the quality of life. Research suggests that following a low FODMAP diet, getting regular exercise, practicing stress management techniques, and taking probiotics may help to reduce symptoms of IBS. Additionally, working with a doctor or health care provider can be beneficial for managing IBS symptoms.

The key to living well with IBS is to find the lifestyle changes that work best for you and make them part of your daily routine. Eating nutritious foods, getting regular physical activity, managing stress levels, and finding emotional support can all be beneficial for helping to manage IBS symptoms. With the right combination of lifestyle changes and medical treatment, it is possible to take control of your symptoms and lead a healthy life.

Irritable Bowel Syndrome Pathophysiology

IBS is caused by changes in the function of the muscles and nerves that control digestion. The digestive tract moves food through the body and absorbs nutrients, but in people with IBS, this process is disrupted. This disruption can result in abdominal pain, bloating, constipation or diarrhoea, and other symptoms.

The exact cause of IBS is unknown, but it is believed to be related to a combination of factors, including genetics, the environment, the immune system, diet, and stress. People with IBS often have an imbalance in their gut bacteria (microbiome) that can lead to increased sensitivity in the digestive tract and changes in the way food moves through the digestive system. Additionally, people with IBS may have an increased sensitivity to certain foods, medications, or hormones.

Research suggests that IBS is a complex disorder with no single cause and that the condition may be triggered by a variety of factors, including stress and diet. Additionally, there is evidence to suggest that people with IBS are more likely to have anxiety and depression, which can further exacerbate their symptoms.

IBS is a chronic condition that has no cure, but with the right combination of lifestyle changes and medical treatment, it is possible to take control of your symptoms and lead a healthy life. Working with a doctor or health care provider can be beneficial for managing IBS symptoms. Additionally, following a low FODMAP diet, getting regular exercise, practicing stress management techniques, and taking probiotics may help to reduce symptoms of IBS.

Ulcerative Colitis

Ulcerative colitis (UC) is an inflammatory bowel disease (IBD) that affects the large intestines of humans. It can cause ulcers and inflammation in the lining of the colon, leading to severe abdominal pain, bloody diarrhoea, fatigue, and weight loss. UC usually responds well to medications and lifestyle changes but may require surgery if symptoms become too severe. Other complications associated with UC include an increased risk of colorectal cancer, arthritis, and eye problems such as uveitis. Early diagnosis and treatment are key to controlling symptoms and keeping the disease in remission.

UC is thought to be caused by a combination of genetic, environmental, and immune factors that interact to lead to inflammation in the colon. While the exact mechanisms are not yet understood, it is believed that an abnormal immune response to bacteria in the colon leads to inflammation and ulceration. Treatment usually focuses on reducing inflammation, preventing complicacions, and managing symptoms.

While there is still much to learn about UC, research has led to improved treatments and new insights into its causes. Understanding how UC works is essential for developing better treatments and finding a cure. With more research, we can help people with UC to manage their symptoms and live healthier lives.

It's important to remember that everyone's experience of UC differs. Some people may have mild symptoms while others may experience severe, disabling disease. Even if treatment helps control your symptoms, it's important to stay informed about the condition and seek support. Talking to a trusted healthcare professional, joining an online community, or finding a local support group can help make living with UC easier.

Ulcerative Colitis Pathophysiology

The pathophysiology of ulcerative colitis involves a complex interplay between inflammatory cells, chemical mediators, and mucosal elements. Inflammation results from an abnormal immune response triggered by the bacteria in the colon. This leads to increased production of pro-inflammatory cytokines as well as other cell signaling molecules which then cause further inflammation.

The inflamed mucosal lining of the colon becomes covered with a thick layer of mucus which leads to ulcers and damaged tissue. This can block nutrients from being absorbed resulting in weight loss, anemia, and other nutrient deficiencies. The damage is progressive and further inflammation occurs as the cycle continues unless it is interrupted by treatment.

Treatment for ulcerative colitis involves using anti-inflammatory medications and immunosuppressants to reduce inflammation, as well as antibiotics to eradicate any infectious agents that may be present. Surgery is sometimes needed if the disease is severe or does not respond to medication. Surgery can involve removing part or all of the colon, with the exact procedure determined by the severity of the patient's symptoms.

While there is still much to learn about the pathophysiology of ulcerative colitis, research has led to new treatments and improved understanding of its causes. With more research, we can continue to develop better treatments for UC and ultimately find a cure. In the meantime, people with UC need to stay informed and seek support when needed.

Gastroesophageal Reflux Disease

Gastroesophageal reflux disease (GERD) is a common digestive disorder that can cause various symptoms such as heartburn, regurgitation, chest pain, and difficulty swallowing. This condition affects mainly the lower oesophagal sphincter, which connects the stomach to the oesophagus. When there is an imbalance in this connection, the stomach acid and contents can travel back up into the oesophagus, causing GERD symptoms. GERD can be managed with lifestyle changes such as avoiding food triggers, eating smaller meals more often, elevating your head while sleeping, and avoiding tight-fitting clothing. Additionally, anti-reflux medications or proton pump inhibitors (PPIs) are commonly used to reduce stomach acid production and improve GERD symptoms. It is important to consult with a healthcare provider if you are experiencing any of these symptoms, as they can help determine the best course of action for your individual needs.

Gastroesophageal Reflux Disease Pathophysiology

The pathophysiology of GERD involves an imbalance between the lower oesophagal sphincter (LES) and the stomach acid. Normally, the LES acts as a barrier that prevents food and stomach acid from flowing back up into the oesophagus. When this balance is disturbed, stomach acid can travel up to the oesophagus, causing GERD symptoms. This can happen due to a variety of factors such as eating large meals, consuming certain foods and beverages, obesity, smoking, alcohol consumption, pregnancy, or taking certain medications. The most common cause is a weakened LES which allows acid reflux from the stomach into the oesophagus.

Gastroesophageal reflux disease can also cause long-term damage to the oesophagus. This is known as "reflux esophagitis" and occurs when stomach acid causes inflammation and irritation of the lining of the oesophagus. Without proper treatment, reflux esophagitis can lead to serious complications such as bleeding, narrowing of the oesophagus, or Barrett's oesophagus, a precancerous condition.

It is important to note that GERD should not be confused with heartburn, which is a symptom of the disorder. Heartburn occurs when stomach acid travels up to and irritates the lining of the oesophagus, causing an uncomfortable burning sensation in the chest or throat. Therefore, if you are experiencing frequent heartburn or any other GERD symptoms, it is important to consult with a healthcare provider for proper diagnosis and treatment.

Peptic Ulcer Disease

Peptic ulcer disease (PUD) is a common medical condition in which ulcers form on the inner lining of the stomach and small intestine. PUD can lead to severe abdominal pain, nausea, bloating, and other digestive symptoms.

The most common cause of peptic ulcer disease is an infection by Helicobacter pylori bacteria. H.

pylori can damage the protective layer of mucus that lines the stomach and small intestine, making it easier for stomach acid to irritate the lining of these organs. Other causes of PUD include long-term use of NSAIDs medications, stress and inflammation.

In addition to medication, lifestyle changes may be recommended as part of the treatment plan for PUD. Eating smaller meals, avoiding spicy food, and limiting or avoiding alcohol consumption can help to alleviate symptoms. Stress management techniques such as relaxation exercises, yoga, and mindfulness meditation may also be beneficial.

It is important to note that peptic ulcer disease is not the same as gastroesophageal reflux disease (GERD). GERD is a condition in which stomach acid backs up into the oesophagus, causing heartburn and other symptoms. However, some people with PUD also have GERD.

Peptic Ulcer Disease Pathophysiology

The pathophysiology of peptic ulcer disease is complex and involves several components. The protective layer of mucus that lines the stomach and small intestine can be damaged by H. pylori, leading to acid exposure that can irritate the lining of these organs. This damage may also result from long-term use of NSAID medications, as well as inflammation and stress.

The damage to the protective layer of mucus leads

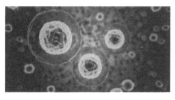 to an increase in gastric acid production, which can further irritate the lining of the stomach and small intestine. In addition, decreased blood flow to these organs can lead to tissue death if not treated promptly. When left untreated, PUD can lead to serious complications such as bleeding from the ulcer site and even perforation of the stomach or small intestine.

In addition, people with PUD are at an increased risk of developing cancer in the digestive tract. This is thought to be due to chronic inflammation caused by H. pylori infection. It is important to seek medical attention if symptoms of PUD persist, as early treatment can help to avoid long-term complications.

Gallstones

Gallstones form when cholesterol or other substances become too concentrated in the gallbladder. These deposits can range in size from a grain of sand to a golf ball and may cause pain, infection, and blockage of bile ducts. Gallstones are more common among women than men, and there is an increased risk for those with a family history of the condition.

Gallstones can form when there is an imbalance in the amount of cholesterol, bilirubin, and bile salts in the gallbladder. This can occur due to factors such as a high-fat diet, weight gain, pregnancy, or certain medications. Additionally, as we age, our gallbladders tend to become less efficient at breaking down cholesterol, which can contribute to gallstone formation.

Gallstones are often asymptomatic, but they can cause a variety of symptoms in some individuals. Symptoms may include abdominal pain, nausea, vomiting, or fever. In severe cases, gallstones can lead to gallbladder inflammation and infection (cholecystitis) or blockage of the common bile duct (choledocholithiasis).

Gallstones Pathophysiology

Gallstones form when there is an excess of cholesterol, bilirubin, and/or bile salts present in the bile. These substances tend to crystalize over time, forming stones known as gallstones. In some cases, the buildup of these substances can cause inflammation and infection in the gallbladder (cholecystitis).

Gallstones can also cause blockage of the common bile duct (choledocholithiasis), which can lead to a cascade of events that may result in severe abdominal pain, jaundice, and pancreatitis. In some cases, gallstones can move from the gallbladder into other parts of the digestive system, such as the small intestine or colon. This is known as gallstone ileus and can cause obstruction of the gastrointestinal tract, leading to abdominal pain and nausea.

If left untreated, gallstones can lead to serious health complications, such as liver damage or pancreatitis. To diagnose gallstones, your doctor may order imaging tests including an ultrasound or CT scan. Treatment options vary depending on the size and number of stones, but may include dietary changes, oral medications, or surgery.

Prevention Of Gallstones

To reduce the risk of developing gallstones, it is important to maintain a healthy lifestyle. Eating a balanced diet that is low in fat and high in fibre can help keep your cholesterol levels under control. Regular exercise can also help regulate your cholesterol levels, as well as reduce your risk of weight gain and obesity. Additionally, it is important to avoid smoking and excessive alcohol consumption.

If you have a family history of gallstones or any other risk factors, it is important to discuss this with your healthcare provider. They can help you identify strategies for preventing or managing the condition. Gallstones can be a serious health concern if left untreated, so it is important to seek medical attention if you think you have symptoms.

Pancreatitis

Pancreatitis is an inflammation of the pancreas, a large organ located behind the stomach which produces enzymes and hormones that aid digestion. It can be acute or chronic and typically presents as abdominal pain, nausea, and vomiting. Acute pancreatitis affects around 5 in every 100,000 people per year, while chronic pancreatitis affects about one in 10,000 people per year.

The most common cause of pancreatitis is gallstone obstruction of the bile ducts which causes an increase in pressure within the pancreas and inflammation. Other causes include high levels of triglycerides, excessive alcohol consumption, drugs or toxins, infections such as mumps virus or HIV, autoimmune disorders like systemic lupus erythematosus, and genetic conditions like cystic fibrosis.

The symptoms of pancreatitis can vary depending on the cause and severity of the inflammation. In acute pancreatitis, patients may experience sudden and severe abdominal pain which is worse after eating or drinking. Other symptoms include nausea and vomiting, fever, rapid heartbeat, jaundice or yellowing of the skin, and rapid breathing. In chronic pancreatitis, patients may experience recurrent abdominal pain as well as nausea, weight loss, diarrhoea or fatty stools, and diabetes.

Pancreatitis Pathophysiology

The pathophysiology of pancreatitis is related to the cause. In acute pancreatitis, inflammation occurs rapidly due to injury or obstruction of the pancreas. This leads to damage and destruction of the pancreatic tissue as well as activation of inflammatory mediators which can result in abdominal pain, fever, and edema in the area surrounding the pancreas.

In chronic pancreatitis, the inflammation is slow and progressive due to repeated injury or obstruction of the pancreas. This leads to scarring of the pancreatic tissue which can interfere with digestive enzyme production and cause abdominal pain as well as other symptoms. Chronic pancreatitis can also lead to diabetes due to decreased insulin production by the pancreas.

Treatment for pancreatitis depends on the cause and severity of the inflammation. Acute pancreatitis is typically treated with supportive care such as intravenous fluids, pain medications, and antibiotics if there is an infection. Chronic pancreatitis may require surgery to remove damaged tissue or the insertion of a stent to keep the bile duct open. Additionally, lifestyle modifications such as quitting smoking, limiting alcohol consumption, and eating a healthy diet are important for managing and preventing the recurrence of pancreatitis.

CHAPTER 7: NEOPLASIA

Neoplasia is the abnormal growth of cells which leads to the formation of tumours. This can be caused by a variety of factors, including genetic mutations and changes in the surrounding environment. Neoplasms can be benign or malignant, with malignant neoplasms being particularly dangerous due to their potential to spread throughout the body and cause further damage. Early detection and treatment are key to successful management of neoplasia. Treatment options include surgery, chemotherapy, and radiation therapy depending on the size, location, and type of tumour present.

Metastasis

Metastasis is the spread of cancer cells from one area of the body to another via circulation or lymphatic vessels. This process can greatly increase the potential severity of a neoplasm and can be difficult to treat due to its ability to spread quickly. Metastatic tumours often occur in distant organs or tissues such as the liver, lungs, brain, and bones and require comprehensive multidisciplinary care for successful management. Treatment options can vary depending on the location of the metastasis but may include chemotherapy, surgery, and radiation.

Early Detection

Early detection of neoplasia is key to successful management and can greatly reduce the risk of spread or recurrence. Regular check-ups with a physician, self-exams for lumps or other changes in size or colour, and blood tests are important ways to monitor changes in the body and early diagnosis is essential for successful treatment. Early detection can also help to reduce the need for more invasive and aggressive treatments such as surgery or radiation therapy.

Neoplasia Pathophysiology

The pathophysiology of neoplasia involves the abnormal growth and division of cells in the body which can be caused by a variety of factors including genetic mutations, changes in the surrounding environment, or exposure to certain toxins or radiation. Neoplasms can originate from any organ or tissue in the body and will generally cause symptoms related to their size and location such as pain, swelling, or changes in function. It is important to seek medical attention if any of these symptoms are present as early diagnosis and treatment can greatly increase the chances of a successful outcome.

Steps Of Neoplasia Pathophysiology

1. Abnormal growth and division of cells

due to genetic mutations, environmental changes, or exposure to certain toxins or radiation.

2. Tumours can be benign or malignant depending on their ability to spread throughout the body.

3. Early detection is key in successful management as it can reduce the potential for metastasis and recurrence.

4. Treatment options such as surgery, chemotherapy, and radiation may be used depending on the size, location, and type of tumour present.

5. Metastasis is the spread of cancer cells from one area to another via circulation or lymphatic vessels which can greatly increase potential severity and difficulty in treatment.

6. Regular check-ups with a physician, self-exams for lumps or other changes in size or colour, and blood tests are important ways to monitor changes in the body.

7. Comprehensive multidisciplinary care is often needed for the successful management of metastasis.

8. Early detection helps reduce the need for more invasive and aggressive treatments such as surgery or radiation therapy.

9. Treatment options vary depending on the location of the metastasis and may include chemotherapy, surgery, and

radiation.

10. Close monitoring of the patient is needed to ensure successful management and reduce the recurrence or spread of neoplasia.

11. Regular check-ups with a physician should be carried out in order to monitor any changes in symptoms or progression of the disease.

12. Supportive therapies such as pain management and nutrition counseling may also be beneficial in managing the symptoms associated with neoplasia.

13. Genetic testing should be considered for family members of those with a diagnosis of neoplasia, as early detection is key to successful treatment.

14. Patients should be made aware of the risks associated with their condition, including the potential for metastasis and recurrence.

15. Regular follow-up visits with a physician are recommended to monitor any changes in symptoms or progression of the disease.

16. Psychological support may also be beneficial for those managing neoplasia as it can help reduce stress and improve quality of life.

17. Further research into the pathophysiology of neoplasia is needed to

better understand the causes and develop more effective treatments.

18. Patients should remain informed about the latest developments in the field as these can help with the successful management of their condition.

19. Nutrition education may be beneficial for those managing neoplasia to help maintain a healthy lifestyle and reduce the risk of recurrence.

20. Complementary therapies such as massage, yoga, and acupuncture may also be beneficial for those managing neoplasia as they can help manage stress and anxiety related to the condition.

Disorders Of The Adrenal Medulla

Adrenal medulla disorders are a group of conditions that affect the body's ability to properly regulate hormones. This can lead to a variety of symptoms and clinical presentations, including high blood pressure, rapid heart rate, fatigue, and sudden weight loss or gain. Disorders of the adrenal medulla may also be caused by tumours or genetic abnormalities. Treatment often involves managing hormone levels through medications and lifestyle changes, such as diet and exercise. If left untreated, these disorders can have serious effects on an individual's health and well-being. It is important to discuss these conditions with your doctor in order to determine the best course of action.

Adrenal medulla hypofunction (also known as Addison's disease) is a condition in which the adrenal gland produces too little of certain hormones. Symptoms can include fatigue, low blood pressure, weight loss, muscle weakness, and darkening of skin colour on exposed areas (such as the face). Treatment involves replacing the missing hormones with medications.

Adrenal medulla hyperfunction (also known as Cushing's syndrome) is a condition in which the adrenal gland produces too much of certain hormones. Symptoms can include weight gain, high blood pressure, and thinning of skin or muscle wasting. Treatment involves controlling hormone levels with medications and lifestyle changes such as diet and exercise.

Adrenal medullary tumours are rare but can cause serious complications if left untreated. The symptoms of these tumours may include weight gain, excessive sweating, and high blood pressure. Treatment usually involves surgically removing the tumour. In some cases, hormone replacement therapy may be necessary.

Finally, genetic disorders can also affect the adrenal medulla and its ability to properly regulate hormones. Symptoms vary depending on the particular disorder, but they often include altered skin colour, rapid heart rate, and abnormal hormone levels. Treatment for these conditions often involves managing the symptoms with medications and lifestyle changes. Genetic disorders can be difficult to diagnose, so it is important to discuss them with your doctor if you are concerned.

Disorders Of The Adrenal Medulla Pathophysiology

The pathophysiology of adrenal medulla disorders varies depending on the particular condition. In cases of adrenal medullary hypofunction, the body is unable to produce sufficient hormones, leading to the symptoms discussed above. On the other hand, in cases of adrenal medullary hyperfunction, the body produces too much of certain hormones, resulting in a different set of symptoms. Adrenal medullary tumours can cause overproduction or underproduction of hormones, depending on the type of tumour. Finally, genetic disorders can alter hormone levels and lead to a variety of symptoms.

In all cases, it is important to seek medical attention as soon as possible in order to determine the best course of treatment for your particular situation. Treatment for adrenal medulla disorders often involves managing the levels of hormones in the body with medications and lifestyle changes. In some cases, surgery may be necessary to remove a tumour or correct a genetic abnormality. It is important to discuss your options with your doctor in order to determine the best course of action for you.

Steps Of Disorders Of The Adrenal Medulla Pathophysiology

The pathophysiology of disorders of the adrenal medulla is a complex process. In general, several steps must occur for these conditions to develop.

First, an underlying cause must be identified, such as a tumour or genetic abnormality. Next, hormone levels in the body become either too high or too low due to the underlying cause. Finally, this leads to a variety of symptoms related to the particular condition that is present.

Once the underlying cause has been identified and treated, hormone levels can usually be managed with medications and lifestyle changes. It is important to follow your doctor's instructions in order to ensure effective treatment and symptom management for your particular situation.

Adrenal medulla disorders can have serious consequences if left untreated, so it is important to seek medical attention as soon as possible. Discussing your symptoms and options with your doctor is the best way to ensure that you receive the most effective treatment for your particular condition.

Disorders Of The Hypothalamus & Pituitary

Gland

There are a variety of disorders that target the hypothalamus and pituitary gland which can lead to increased morbidity or mortality. These disorders include benign tumours, malignant tumours, craniopharyngiomas, congenital hypothyroidism, hyperprolactinemia, Cushing's Disease, Addison's Disease and acromegaly.

Benign tumours are non-cancerous growths that can cause hormonal imbalances and can lead to vision loss if they occur near the optic chiasm. Malignant tumours are cancerous growths that have the potential of invading surrounding tissue and organs, making early detection crucial for successful treatment. Craniopharyngiomas are benign tumours that form near the pituitary gland and can cause hypothalamic dysfunction, which can lead to the failure of growth hormone secretion.

Congenital hypothyroidism is a disorder caused by an underactive thyroid gland due to insufficient levels of thyroid hormones. Symptoms include mental retardation, stunted growth, delayed puberty and abnormal development of organs and tissues. Hyperprolactinemia is an excessive amount of the hormone prolactin that can cause infertility, headaches, and irregular menstrual cycles.

Cushing's Disease is caused by high levels of

cortisol hormones due to a pituitary gland disorder. Symptoms include osteoporosis, weight gain, fatigue and weak muscles. Addison's Disease is caused by a lack of the hormones cortisol and aldosterone. Common symptoms include fatigue, weight loss, muscle weakness and salt cravings. Acromegaly is caused by an overproduction of growth hormone due to either a benign pituitary tumour or excessive stimulation from another hormone-releasing tumour elsewhere in the body. Symptoms include enlargement of hands, feet and facial bones, excessive sweating and headaches.

It is important to understand the various types of disorders that can affect the hypothalamus and pituitary gland in order to detect them early on and provide necessary treatment. Early diagnosis and treatment of these conditions can help improve quality of life, reduce morbidity and mortality rates, and prevent long-term complications.

Disorders Of The Hypothalamus & Pituitary Gland Pathophysiology

In order to understand the pathologic processes of these disorders, it is important to examine the anatomy and physiology of the hypothalamus and pituitary gland. The hypothalamus serves as an endocrine organ that regulates water balance, temperature regulation, hunger, behaviour and hormone production. It is also responsible for regulating the release of hormones from the pituitary gland. The pituitary gland is divided into two distinct parts; the anterior lobe and the posterior lobe. The anterior lobe produces many hormones, including growth hormone, adrenocorticotropic hormone (ACTH) and thyroid-stimulating hormone (TSH). The posterior lobe produces antidiuretic hormone (ADH), oxytocin and endorphins.

Steps Of Disorders Of The Hypothalamus & Pituitary Gland Pathophysiology

Disorders of the hypothalamus and pituitary gland can arise from many different sources, including genetic mutations, environmental factors or infections. Disorders can occur due to a decrease in hormone production, an increase in hormone production or due to a structural change in the gland itself.

The first step in diagnosing a disorder is for physicians to determine the source of the hormonal imbalance and to determine what hormone levels are affected. This involves taking a thorough medical history, performing physical exams, assessing symptoms and ordering blood tests or imaging studies.

Once the source of the disorder is identified, physicians can use medications or other treatments to restore normal hormone production or reduce the size of a tumour. Surgery may be necessary for certain types of tumours, while radiation therapy or chemotherapy may be used to treat malignant tumours.

People with disorders of the hypothalamus and pituitary gland need to receive regular follow-up care in order to monitor symptoms and adjust treatment as needed. Long-term complications can include vision loss, infertility, nerve damage and other issues that can greatly impact the quality of life. Therefore, it is important to receive proper diagnosis and treatment for these conditions in order to avoid long-term complications.

Sleep Apnea

Sleep Apnea is a condition wherein breathing is interrupted during sleep. It results from the collapse of the upper airways due to muscle relaxation or obstruction, causing an individual to stop breathing for several seconds multiple times a night. These pauses in breathing can occur up to 30 times per hour and may last anywhere from 10-20 seconds. This can cause a decrease in the oxygen levels in the body, leading to further health issues.

Sleep Apnea can lead to insomnia as well as other sleep-related disorders such as snoring and restless legs syndrome. Additionally, it can cause fatigue during waking hours, difficulty concentrating, and an overall feeling of tiredness.

People with Sleep Apnea are also at risk for more serious health problems such as high blood pressure, heart disease, diabetes, and stroke.

It is important to seek medical help for this condition as it can lead to further health issues if left untreated. Treatment options may include lifestyle modification such as losing weight or stopping smoking, as well as the use of specialized devices like Continuous Positive Airway Pressure (CPAP) machines. In some cases, surgery may be recommended to remove blockages in the airways that are causing Sleep Apnea.

Steps Of Sleep Apnea Pathophysiology

1. Relaxation of airway muscles – During sleep, the muscles in the upper throat relax, which can cause them to collapse onto the walls of the throat. This narrows the upper airways and leads to a reduction in airflow.

2. Obstruction of the Airways - An obstruction in the airways can also occur due to an enlarged tongue or tonsils, leading to further narrowing of the airways.

3. Decreased Oxygen Levels - As a result of airway obstruction, oxygen levels in the body can decrease due to a lack of airflow. This can be dangerous, as it can lead to further health issues such as high blood

pressure and stroke.

4. Respiratory Arrest – In some cases, the decreased oxygen levels can lead to a complete stop in breathing for several seconds. This is known as Respiratory Arrest and is a dangerous condition.

5. Restlessness - Although the body is attempting to resume normal breathing patterns, this may be difficult due to the obstruction of the airways and could cause restlessness during sleep.

6. Daytime Symptoms - As a result of sleep disruptions and decreased oxygen levels, people with Sleep Apnea often experience daytime symptoms such as fatigue, difficulty concentrating, and an overall feeling of tiredness.

Lung Cancer

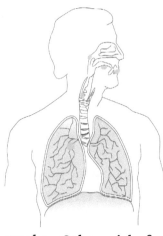

Lung cancer is the leading cause of cancer-related death in both men and women in the United States. While there are many types of lung cancers, most cases are caused by smoking cigarettes or exposure to other forms of tobacco smoke. Other risk factors for developing lung cancer include air pollution, radiation therapy, family history, and occupational exposure to carcinogens.

The most common type of lung cancer is non-small cell lung cancer (NSCLC). NSCLC accounts for about 80% of all cases and is usually treated with chemotherapy and radiation. Small cell lung cancer (SCLC) accounts for the remaining 20% of cases and is more aggressive, typically requiring treatment with chemotherapy or radiation in combination with surgery.

The prognosis for lung cancer depends on the stage of the disease at the time of diagnosis. If caught early, there is a better chance of successful treatment and survival. However, if lung cancer has spread to other parts of the body, it can be more difficult to treat and may require more aggressive therapy such as immunotherapy or targeted drug therapy.

No matter what type of lung cancer a patient has, it is important to monitor the disease for signs of progression and adjust treatment accordingly. While there are no known cures for lung cancer, advances in treatment have led to improved outcomes for many patients.

Lung Cancer Pathophysiology

Lung cancer pathogenesis is a complex process that involves genetic and environmental factors, including both oncogenic mutations in DNA and exposure to carcinogens. Oncogenic mutations can occur naturally through the ageing process or from inherited gene defects, but they are also associated with smoking cigarettes or other forms of tobacco smoke. These mutations can lead to uncontrolled cell proliferation and tumour formation.

Environmental factors like air pollution, radiation therapy, and occupational exposure to carcinogens can also contribute to the development of lung cancer. These factors can cause DNA damage that results in mutations and uncontrolled cell proliferation.

In addition to genetic and environmental factors, some individuals may be more susceptible to developing lung cancer due to certain risk factors. These include a family history of lung cancer, being older than 65 years old, having a weakened immune system, and having certain chronic medical conditions such as COPD or asthma.

Steps Of Lung Cancer Pathophysiology

The pathogenesis of lung cancer involves several steps. The first step is the initiation phase, which is when genetic mutations occur in cells due to environmental factors or inherited gene defects. These mutations can lead to uncontrolled cell proliferation and tumour formation.

The second step is the promotion phase, where changes in cell structure and function lead to the growth of tumours. This can be caused by both genetic and environmental factors.

The third step is the progression phase, which is when tumours become more malignant and spread to other parts of the body. During this phase, there may also be changes in gene expression that lead to further tumour growth and metastasis.

Finally, the fourth step is the metastatic phase where cancer cells metastasize, or spread, to other organs in the body. This is typically the most advanced stage of lung cancer and can be difficult to treat.

Tissue Damage

Tissue damage occurs when tissue is subjected to injuries or illnesses that cause it to malfunction or die. Damage can be caused by a variety of factors, including physical trauma, chemical burns, radiation exposure, environmental toxins, and certain medical conditions. Depending on the type and extent of the injury or illness, tissue may be damaged immediately or over time.

Tissue damage can lead to inflammation, pain, scarring, and in some cases cell death. It can also cause complications such as tissue necrosis (tissue death), infection, and an increased risk of developing cancer. In severe cases, tissue damage may end up needing surgery or organ transplantation in order to repair the damaged area.

When tissue damage occurs, the body's immune system is activated to help repair and heal it. The immune response helps reduce inflammation, as well as produce substances that promote healing. In some cases, medications can be prescribed to help reduce pain and swelling associated with tissue damage.

Tissue Damage Pathophysiology

The pathophysiology of tissue damage involves the processes and reactions that occur when tissue is damaged. These changes can be seen both at a cellular and molecular level, as well as in the tissues' overall structure and function.

At a cellular level, damage to cells causes disruption of their normal functioning. This disruption can manifest itself as a decrease in energy production, increased levels of cellular debris, and the release of various chemical mediators such as cytokines that can further damage surrounding tissues.

Molecular changes to damaged cells can include changes in gene expression and the activation of pathways which lead to cell death. This process is known as apoptosis. Apoptosis is a process by which cells are destroyed in an orderly fashion, and the body must rid itself of damaged or unwanted cells.

At the tissue level, damage can lead to

inflammation, reduced blood flow, and scarring. These changes often result in altered cell function and structure. They can also lead to further disruption of normal tissue architecture, increased risk of infection, and long-term complications such as organ failure.

Pathophysiology of tissue damage is a complex process that involves multiple layers of interactions between cells, tissues, organs, and the environment. Understanding the various components and how they interact is essential to understanding how tissue damage occurs and how best to treat it.

Steps Of Tissue Damage Pathophysiology

The pathophysiology of tissue damage begins when the body is exposed to an external injury or illness. This can be a physical trauma, chemical burn, radiation exposure, environmental toxin, or medical condition. The initial event triggers various physiological responses from the body that lead to inflammation and tissue damage.

The inflammatory process causes swelling and pain in the affected area, and it can lead to further tissue damage. In some cases, the inflammation causes cells in the area to die due to a lack of oxygen or nutrients. This process is known as necrosis.

The body then begins a healing process by activating its immune system and sending signaling molecules such as cytokines that help repair damaged tissues. At this stage, medications may be prescribed to help reduce inflammation and pain.

The body then begins to rebuild the damaged tissue by forming new connective tissues and regenerating cells. This process can take weeks or months depending on the type of injury, and it can be complicated by infection of the area, scarring, or organ failure.

Tissue damage pathophysiology involves multiple layers of complexity, and understanding the process is essential for effective treatment and prevention of tissue damage. With a greater understanding of pathophysiology, doctors and researchers are able to develop better treatments for tissue damage. In addition, preventive measures such as avoiding exposure to toxins or radiation can help reduce the risk of tissue damage in the first place.

Prevention and awareness of tissue damage pathophysiology are key to reducing the incidence and severity of tissue damage. By understanding the various elements and processes involved in tissue damage, healthcare providers can better diagnose, treat, and prevent it.

The understanding of tissue damage pathophysiology can also help researchers develop new treatments for tissue injuries and illnesses. With greater knowledge of the process, researchers can develop more effective strategies for healing and preventing tissue damage.

The pathophysiology of tissue damage is a complex process, but with a greater understanding of the various components involved, healthcare providers and researchers can effectively diagnose, treat, and prevent it. Awareness and prevention are key to reducing the incidence of tissue damage, as well as developing treatments that help restore damaged tissues and organs.

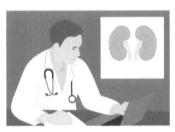

Chronic Kidney Disease

Chronic kidney disease (CKD) is a term that describes the gradual decline in kidney function over time. The kidneys are two bean-shaped organs located in the upper abdomen, one on each side of the spine, which serve to filter waste and other substances from the body. When CKD develops, these filtering functions become impaired.

The causes of CKD can be divided into two broad categories: primary and secondary. Primary kidney disease is caused by direct damage to the kidneys, such as through infection or injury. Secondary kidney disease occurs when another condition or disease affects the kidneys, for example, high blood pressure or diabetes.

Signs and symptoms of CKD include tiredness, swelling in the face and extremities, decreased appetite, nausea, and weight loss. Other symptoms may include changes in urine output or colour, foamy urine, and dark circles under the eyes. As CKD progresses, it can cause other complications such as heart disease, anaemia, bone disease (osteoporosis), nerve damage (peripheral neuropathy), and even kidney failure.

Chronic Kidney Disease Pathophysiology

The pathophysiology of CKD can vary depending on the cause. In general, impaired kidney function can be caused by damage to the glomeruli (filtering units in kidneys) or by changes in blood flow through the kidneys. In addition, systemic inflammation and damage to the tubules (tiny tubes that transport fluid from within the kidneys) can also contribute to the pathophysiology of CKD.

When the glomeruli are damaged, they can no longer filter waste efficiently and cause toxins to build up in the body. The buildup of toxins can lead to a number of symptoms such as fatigue, nausea, weight loss, and anaemia. Additionally, when the tubules are damaged it affects how well fluids are transported in and out of the kidneys, leading to swelling in the face and extremities.

CKD has a number of serious complications

that can arise from long-term deterioration of kidney function. These include metabolic acidosis, anaemia, electrolyte imbalance, hypertension, heart disease, bone disease (osteoporosis), nerve damage (peripheral neuropathy), and even kidney failure.

Early detection and treatment of CKD are critical to managing the condition and can help reduce the risk of complications. Treatment typically involves controlling underlying conditions such as high blood pressure or diabetes, lifestyle modifications (e.g., diet, exercise), medications, and dialysis therapy for end-stage renal disease. Regular checkups with a healthcare provider are important to ensure that the condition is being monitored and treated appropriately.

By recognizing the signs and symptoms of CKD early, people can take steps to protect their kidneys and reduce their risk of complications. With proper monitoring and treatment, many people with CKD can enjoy a full life despite their diagnosis.

Steps Of Chronic Kidney Disease Pathophysiology

1. Damage to the glomeruli leads to reduced filtration of waste, and toxins begin to accumulate in the body, leading to a range of symptoms.

2. Damage to the tubules affects how fluids are transported in and out of the kidneys, leading to swelling in the face and extremities.
3. Long-term deterioration of kidney function can lead to a number of serious complications, including metabolic acidosis, anaemia, hypertension, heart disease and even kidney failure.
4. Early detection and treatment are important for managing CKD and can help reduce the risk of complications.
5. With proper monitoring and treatment, many people with CKD can enjoy a full life despite their diagnosis.
6. Making healthy lifestyle changes, such as eating a balanced diet and exercising regularly, can help reduce the risk of CKD progression.
7. Regular checkups with a doctor are important for monitoring kidney function and ensuring that any complications or potential issues are caught early on.

Cystic Fibrosis Patients

Cystic fibrosis (CF) is a genetic disorder that affects the respiratory and digestive systems in children and adults. It is caused by a mutation in the cystic fibrosis transmembrane conductance regulator (CFTR) gene, resulting in thick mucus buildup which clogs the airways, leading to increased lung infections. Additionally, it can lead to a decreased absorption of nutrients in the intestines, resulting in malnutrition and weight loss.

Due to the buildup of thick mucus, cystic fibrosis patients experience respiratory symptoms such as coughing, wheezing, shortness of breath, and lung infections. Gastrointestinal problems like constipation, diarrhoea, gas and bloating are also common. Additionally, cystic fibrosis patients often experience fatigue, delayed growth, and difficulty gaining weight.

Cystic Fibrosis Patients Pathophysiology

The main pathophysiology of cystic fibrosis is due to the mutation in the CFTR gene. This results in a buildup of thick mucus, which clogs the airways and affects multiple organs. The mucus buildup also increases susceptibility to bacterial infections, leading to increased lung infections and inflammation. Additionally, it causes damage to other organs such as the pancreas, which can lead to poor absorption of nutrients.

The thick mucus buildup in the lungs and airways causes difficulty breathing and often requires frequent treatments with antibiotics, bronchodilators, and other medications. The mucus buildup also increases susceptibility to bacterial infections, leading to increased lung infections and inflammation. In addition, cystic fibrosis patients may experience malnutrition due to the decreased absorption of nutrients in the intestines.

Steps Of Cystic Fibrosis Patients Pathophysiology

The main treatment for cystic fibrosis is to help manage the symptoms and slow down the progression of the disease. Treatment plans are typically tailored to each individual patient, depending on their age, activity level, lifestyle, health goals, and other factors. The primary goal of treatment is to improve lung function and reduce the risk of infection.

To reduce the risk of infection, cystic fibrosis patients are encouraged to get regular vaccinations and practice good hygiene. They may also need to take antibiotics to treat bacterial infections or use inhaled medications or bronchodilators to help open their airways and ease breathing difficulties.

Nutritional therapy is also an important part of cystic fibrosis treatment, as it helps to ensure that patients get the proper nutrients they need to stay healthy. This may involve taking nutritional supplements or eating a high-calorie diet with lots of fruits, vegetables, and lean proteins. Exercise is also an important part of managing cystic fibrosis and can help improve lung function.

Finally, emotional support and lifestyle changes

are often key components of managing cystic fibrosis. Patients need to be aware of the risks associated with the disease and take steps to minimize them, such as avoiding cigarette smoke and dust. They should also find a support system of family and friends who can help provide emotional support when needed. By following these steps, cystic fibrosis patients can often improve their quality of life and reduce symptoms of the disease.

CHAPTER 8: NEURODEGENERATIVE DISEASES

N eurodegenerative diseases are conditions that cause progressive degeneration and/ or death of neurons, which are the cells in your brain and body that transmit communication signals between one another. This type of disease can have a wide range of causes including genetic conditions, environmental factors or aging-related changes. Symptoms may vary but common signs include memory loss, difficulty finding words, difficulty with balance and coordination, and mood changes. The most common forms of neurodegenerative diseases are Alzheimer's disease, Parkinson's disease, Huntington's disease, Lou Gehrig's (Amyotrophic Lateral Sclerosis) and Multiple Sclerosis.

Alzheimer's Disease

Alzheimer's disease is a progressive and irreversible neurological disorder that affects memory, language, and behaviour. It is the most common form of dementia, accounting for 60-80% of all cases. The cause of Alzheimer's disease is not yet known but risk factors include age, family history, and genetics.

Symptoms can range from mild memory loss to severe cognitive decline. Common symptoms include difficulty with memory, word-finding and language; changes in behaviour or personality; difficulty with planning and organizing; confusion about time and place; and difficulty completing familiar tasks. As Alzheimer's progresses, people may experience increased apathy, aggression, delusions and hallucinations, sleep disturbances, incontinence, and problems with walking and balance.

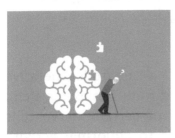

Alzheimer's Disease Pathophysiology

Alzheimer's disease is characterized by the accumulation of two types of lesions in the brain: amyloid plaques and neurofibrillary tangles. Amyloid plaques are deposits of a protein called beta-amyloid, which form outside nerve cells and interfere with their function. Neurofibrillary tangles are composed of a protein called tau, which forms inside nerve cells and disrupt their ability to communicate with each other. In addition, inflammation is believed to play an important role in the development of Alzheimer's disease.

Alzheimer's disease pathophysiology is complex and not fully understood. Recent research suggests that changes in the brain begin decades before symptoms appear, suggesting that there may be treatments available to slow or even prevent the disease.

Currently, there is no cure for Alzheimer's disease, but treatments are available to help manage symptoms and improve quality of life. These include medications to improve cognition and reduce behavioural problems; psychological therapies; support groups; and lifestyle changes such as exercise and sleep hygiene. Research into treatments that target the underlying cause of Alzheimer's disease is ongoing.

Parkinson's Disease

Parkinson's disease is a neurodegenerative disorder that affects the brain and nervous system. It is caused by the loss of certain nerve cells in the brain, which leads to abnormal activity in parts of the brain associated with movement control. Symptoms include stiffness, tremors, slowed movement, and difficulty with balance and coordination.

The exact cause of Parkinson's disease is still unknown, but researchers believe it could be due to genetic and environmental factors. Research has shown that people with certain genetic mutations are more likely to develop Parkinson's, while exposure to chemicals or toxins can increase the risk of developing the disorder.

Parkinson's Disease Pathophysiology

The pathophysiology of Parkinson's disease involves the destruction or malfunction of neurons in the brain. Specifically, cells in a region called the substantia nigra (SN) are damaged or destroyed, leading to reduced levels of dopamine in certain areas of the brain. This disruption causes symptoms such as slowness of movement and difficulty with coordination and balance.

The other area of the brain affected by Parkinson's is the striatum, which receives signals from the SN and helps to control movement. When dopamine levels in this area are impaired, it can lead to an inability to move or initiate movement. Other symptoms, such as tremors, may also occur due to decreased activity in different parts of the basal ganglia.

In addition to the physical symptoms, Parkinson's disease can also have an impact on mental health. People with the disorder may experience depression, anxiety, and other psychiatric disorders. As the disease progresses, cognitive decline can be observed due to nerve cell death in areas of the brain related to memory and thinking.

Steps Of Parkinson's Disease Pathophysiology

1. Neurons in the substantia nigra (SN) are damaged or destroyed, leading to reduced levels of dopamine in certain areas of the brain.
2. This disruption causes symptoms such as slowness of movement and difficulty

with coordination and balance.

3. The striatum is also affected by Parkinson's, receiving signals from the SN and helping to control movement.

4. When dopamine levels in this area are impaired, it can lead to an inability to move or initiate movement, as well as tremors.

5. Parkinson's disease can also have an impact on mental health, leading to depression, anxiety, and other psychiatric disorders.

6. As the disease progresses, cognitive decline can be observed due to nerve cell death in areas of the brain related to memory and thinking.

7. Treatment options for Parkinson's disease include medications, surgery, physical therapy, and lifestyle changes.

8. While there is no cure for Parkinson's disease, these treatments can help manage symptoms and improve quality of life.

By understanding the underlying pathophysiology of Parkinson's disease, healthcare providers can develop more effective treatment plans to help slow the progression of the disorder and improve quality of life. With continued research, we can someday find a cure for this devastating illness.

Prevention

Although there is no sure way to prevent Parkinson's disease, it is possible to reduce your risk by making lifestyle changes and avoiding certain chemicals or toxins. Eating a healthy diet, staying physically active, and getting enough rest can help to reduce the risk of neurological disorders such as Parkinson's. Additionally, avoiding exposure to toxic chemicals in the workplace or at home is also important for reducing the risk of developing this disorder.

Huntington's Disease

Huntington's disease (HD) is an inherited genetic disorder affecting the brain. It affects people of all ages, genders, and ethnic backgrounds. HD is caused by a mutation in the huntingtin gene which results in a gradual decline in cognitive function over time. Symptoms of HD may include muscular jerking movements (called chorea), difficulty walking, speaking, and swallowing difficulty, changes in behaviour and personality, and progressive dementia.

HD is a slowly progressing disorder that has no cure. Treatment focuses on managing the symptoms of HD to improve the quality of life for those affected. This may include medications, speech/physical/ occupational therapy, psychological counseling, lifestyle modifications such as a healthy diet and regular exercise, and supportive care such as respite care.

HD is a difficult disease to diagnose because the symptoms can be similar to other neurological diseases. It is important for people who may be at risk of HD to see their doctor for testing and evaluation if they notice any of its early signs or symptoms, or if there is a family history of HD. Early diagnosis and intervention can help reduce the progression of HD, as well as provide support for those affected.

Huntington's Disease Pathophysiology

The pathophysiology of HD is complex and still being studied. The mutation in the huntingtin gene results in excessive amounts of the protein Huntingtin (Htt) which accumulates in neurons and causes them to be dysfunctional or die. This damage leads to gradual changes in a person's behaviour, motor skills, cognitive function, and emotional state associated with HD.

Damage to the brain's circuits affects multiple areas of the brain, which has a domino effect throughout the body. The damage done by HD may cause problems with movement control, speech and language processing, memory and learning, as well as emotional regulation. These problems can lead to physical and mental exhaustion, reduced ability to care for oneself, difficulty communicating with others, and depression.

HD is a progressive disorder that can affect

people differently, so it is important to work with healthcare professionals to develop an individualized treatment plan tailored to the needs of each person. Such plans may include medications, physical therapy, speech/language therapy, psychological counseling, lifestyle modifications such as diet and exercise, and supportive care such as respite care.

Steps Of Huntington's Disease Pathophysiology

1. The mutation in the huntingtin gene codes for an abnormally large, abnormal form of the protein Huntingtin (Htt).
2. The Htt accumulates in neurons and is toxic to them, leading to progressive cell death throughout the brain over time.
3. This neuronal damage disrupts the function of multiple areas of the brain, including those responsible for movement control, speech/language processing, memory and learning, and emotional regulation.
4. Over time, these disruptions result in the physical and psychological changes associated with HD such as chorea, difficulty walking, speaking and swallowing difficulty, changes in behavior and personality, and progressive dementia.
5. Early diagnosis of HD is important so that

individuals can receive treatment and management of symptoms sooner, which can help reduce the progression of HD.

6. Treatment plans for HD may include medications, physical/speech/language therapy, psychological counseling, lifestyle modifications such as diet and exercise, and supportive care such as respite care.

7. These treatments are aimed at improving quality of life for those affected by HD and slowing the progression of the disorder.

8. Research is ongoing to find new treatments for HD and improve existing ones.

9. Support groups and organizations dedicated to helping those with HD can also provide emotional support, education, and access to resources for individuals affected by HD and their families.

10. HD is a lifelong condition and it is important to continue to receive care and support throughout its progression.

11. Working with healthcare professionals, individuals affected by HD can develop an individualized care plan that takes into account their own needs as well as the latest research on treatment options for managing symptoms of the disorder.

12. It is also important for individuals to

take steps to maintain their physical and mental health, such as engaging in regular exercise and healthy eating.

13. Having a strong support network of family and friends can also be beneficial in helping individuals cope with the challenges posed by HD.

Amyotrophic Lateral Sclerosis

Amyotrophic lateral sclerosis (ALS) is a progressive neurological condition that affects the motor neurons in the brain and spinal cord, leading to muscle weakness and wasting. In ALS, nerve cells gradually lose their ability to send signals to the muscles, causing them to stop working properly. As the disease progresses, patients often experience difficulty with everyday tasks such as walking, speaking, and swallowing. In advanced cases of ALS, the condition can lead to respiratory failure.

The cause of ALS is not completely understood, but research suggests that a combination of genetic and environmental factors may be involved. Some studies have found an association between military service and an increased risk of developing ALS later in life, although the exact connection remains unclear. Additionally, while there is no known cure for ALS, medications and other treatments can help manage the symptoms and improve quality of life. Physical therapy, occupational therapy, speech-language pathology, respiratory therapy, nutritional counseling, and psychological support are all important components of an ALS treatment plan. With proper care and support from family and friends, people living with ALS can have a better overall quality of life.

While ALS is a debilitating condition, advances in research have improved the outlook for people living with ALS. In particular, stem cell therapy has been shown to be effective in improving muscle strength and functionality in some cases. Additionally, research into gene therapy and other experimental treatments show promising results for slowing the progression of the disease. With continued progress in understanding how to treat ALS, patients have hope for living longer and better lives with the condition.

Amyotrophic Lateral Sclerosis Pathophysiology

Pathophysiologically, ALS is a progressive neurodegenerative disorder in which nerve cells in the brain and spinal cord are gradually lost. As these cells decline, their ability to send signals to muscles decreases, leading to muscle weakness and wasting. The exact cause of this degeneration remains unknown, although some evidence suggests that genetic mutations may play a role. Additionally, environmental factors such as exposure to certain toxins or radiation may be involved.

There is no known cure for ALS, but treatments are available to help manage symptoms and improve quality of life. Physical therapy and occupational therapy can help maintain muscle strength and function, while speech-language pathology can reduce the effects of speech impairment. Additionally, nutritional counseling and respiratory therapy can help patients cope with difficulties in breathing and eating. Psychological support can also provide important assistance to those living with ALS, helping them to cope with the emotional and social challenges of the disease.

As research continues into treatments for ALS, promising new therapies show promise for slowing progression of the condition. In particular, stem cell therapy has been found to be effective in improving muscle strength and functionality in some cases. Additionally, research into gene therapy and other experimental treatments offer the potential for improved diagnosis and treatment of ALS. With continued progress in understanding how to treat ALS, those affected can find hope for living longer and better lives with the condition.

Steps Of Amyotrophic Lateral Sclerosis Pathophysiology

1. Damage to the motor neurons in the brain and spinal cord leads to difficulty sending signals to muscles, causing them to become weak and waste away.
2. The exact cause of this degeneration is unknown, although genetic mutations and environmental factors may play a role.
3. There is no known cure for ALS, but treatments are available to help manage symptoms and improve quality of life.
4. Physical therapy, occupational therapy, speech-language pathology, respiratory therapy, nutritional counseling and psychological support can all be important components of an ALS treatment plan.
5. Stem cell therapy has been found to be effective in improving muscle strength and functionality in some cases while research into gene therapy and other experimental treatments offer the potential for improved diagnosis and treatment of ALS.
6. With continued progress in understanding how to treat ALS, those affected can find hope for living longer and better lives with the condition.

Mood Disorder

Mood disorders, also known as affective disorders, are a category of mental health disorders that involve distorted or extreme shifts in mood. These can include depression (major depressive disorder) and bipolar disorder, which is characterized by alternating periods of mania and depression. Mood swings associated with these conditions can range from mild to severe in intensity.

Common signs and symptoms of mood disorders include persistent sadness, feelings of emptiness or hopelessness, anxiety, changes in appetite or sleep patterns, restlessness or irritability, low energy levels, poor concentration or memory problems, and thoughts of death or suicide.

Mood Disorder Pathophysiology

Mood disorders involve disruptions in the body's natural internal balance of neurotransmitters, hormones, and other chemicals that help regulate mood. Neurotransmitters — chemical messengers in the brain that are involved in regulating mood — can be affected by factors such as stress, illness, genetics, or changes in hormone levels.

It is believed that brain abnormalities can also play a role in the development of mood disorders. Studies have suggested that specific parts of the brain involved in regulating emotions may be larger or smaller than normal in people with mood disorders.

Furthermore, changes to areas of the brain

responsible for reward processing and decision-making can lead to difficulty controlling impulses, which may further contribute to these conditions.

The exact pathophysiology of mood disorders is not fully understood, and more research is needed in this area. However, it is clear that a combination of genetic, environmental, and neurological factors contribute to the development of these conditions. Treatment typically involves a combination of psychotherapy and medications such as antidepressants or mood stabilizers. It is important to note that each person's experience with mood disorders is unique, and the most effective treatment plan should be tailored to one's individual needs.

Treatment Of Mood Disorders

Treatment options for mood disorders vary depending on the severity and type of disorder. Generally, treatment plans focus on improving a person's ability to cope with symptoms and helping them develop skills that can reduce the intensity and frequency of episodes.

Psychotherapy is an effective approach for managing mood disorders, and may involve techniques such as cognitive-behavioral therapy (CBT), dialectical behavior therapy (DBT), and interpersonal psychotherapy (IPT). These types of therapy focus on helping people identify patterns in their thoughts and behaviors that contribute to their disorder, develop healthy coping skills, and recognize triggers that can lead to episodes.

Medications may also be prescribed in combination with psychotherapy to improve symptoms of mood disorders. Antidepressants are commonly used to treat depression, while antipsychotics and mood stabilizers are often prescribed for bipolar disorder. It is important to remember that medications may take several weeks or more before they have any effect, and it may take time to find the right medication and dosage.

In some cases, electroconvulsive therapy (ECT) may be recommended for severe depression that is unresponsive to medications or psychotherapy. This treatment involves passing small electrical currents through the brain to induce seizures which can help reset the neurological pathways in the brain.

Depression Disorder

Depression is a serious mental health disorder caused by an imbalance in the brain's neurotransmitters, including dopamine, serotonin, and norepinephrine. It is characterized by persistent feelings of sadness and hopelessness that can affect daily life activities such as sleeping, eating, and concentration. Common symptoms include fatigue, insomnia, lack of interest in activities, difficulty concentrating, and suicidal thoughts. Treatment for depression usually consists of psychotherapy, medications, or a combination of both. Medications such as antidepressants can help regulate the brain's neurotransmitters to improve mood and reduce symptoms of depression. Psychotherapy can also be beneficial in helping individuals understand their thoughts and feelings about themselves and their life experiences. By understanding these feelings, they can find more constructive ways to cope and move forward. It is important for individuals with depression to seek help from a mental health professional, as depression can be debilitating and even life-threatening if left untreated. With the right support and treatment, those living with depression can lead healthy and fulfilling lives.

Depression disorder affects many aspects of an individual's functioning. Those struggling with depression may experience difficulty in their relationships, work, and leisure activities. They may have trouble sleeping or concentrating on tasks, as well as feel isolated from others. They can also experience physical symptoms such as headaches and muscle tension.

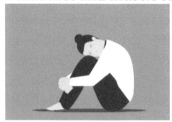

Depression Disorder Pathophysiology

The exact causes of depression disorder are

not fully understood. However, research has shown that there is likely a combination of genetic, biological, environmental, and psychological factors at play. Biological factors may include an imbalance in neurotransmitters, such as serotonin and norepinephrine, which can lead to changes in mood. Genetic predisposition also appears to be involved in some cases, and environmental factors like stress or a traumatic event can also be contributing factors. It is important for individuals to understand the different aspects that can contribute to depression in order to better manage and treat it.

Research has also suggested that inflammation may play an important role in depression disorder. Inflammation occurs when your body's immune system releases chemicals in response to infection or injury. This immune response can lead to increased levels of inflammatory proteins in the body, which may be linked to symptoms of depression. Additionally, stress hormones such as cortisol and epinephrine can disrupt your brain's natural balance and contribute to feelings of anxiety and depression.

Depression disorder is a serious condition that requires treatment from a mental health professional. Treatment may involve psychotherapy, medications, or a combination of both in order to reduce symptoms and improve functioning. Individuals with depression disorder need to seek help from a mental health professional and create an individualized treatment plan that fits their needs. With the right support and treatment, those living with depression can lead healthy and fulfilling lives.

It is important to note that depression disorder is not necessarily a sign of weakness or lack of will power. It is a serious condition that requires medical attention and should be discussed with a mental health professional. With the right support and treatment, those living with depression can lead healthy and fulfilling lives.

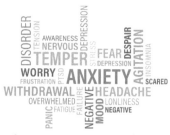

Anxiety Disorders

Anxiety disorders are a group of mental health conditions that are characterized by fear, worry, and uneasiness. These can range from mild to severe and may include physical symptoms such as sweating, trembling, or nausea. Anxiety can impact one's daily life by causing difficulties in concentration and sleeping patterns as well as leading to avoidance behaviors.

There are many different types of anxiety disorders, such as generalized anxiety disorder (GAD), panic disorder, and social anxiety disorder. Treatment typically involves talk therapy or medication depending on the severity of symptoms. Research is being done to better understand how genetics, environmental factors, and psychological factors can all contribute to the development of an anxiety disorder.

Self-care strategies such as relaxation and mindfulness techniques can be used to help manage symptoms of anxiety. Additionally, lifestyle changes such as reducing alcohol and caffeine intake or getting more regular exercise may also be beneficial in managing anxiety. Seeking professional help from a mental health provider is also encouraged if symptoms persist or worsen over time.

Anxiety Disorders Pathophysiology

The exact causes of anxiety disorders are not yet fully understood, but they likely involve a combination of genetic, environmental, and psychological factors. Genetics plays a role in the development of anxiety disorders since they tend to be more common among people who have a family history of such conditions. Environmental factors can also contribute to the development of an anxiety disorder. Trauma, abuse, and other stressful life events can increase one's risk of developing an anxiety disorder. Psychological factors such as a person's personality traits or learned behaviors can also be involved in the development of an anxiety disorder.

It is thought that people with anxiety disorders

have changes to certain areas of the brain, which results in a different type of brain activity. For example, those with panic disorder may have an overactive amygdala, which leads to increased fear and anxiety in response to perceived threats. Furthermore, research has suggested that people with anxiety disorders often have higher levels of cortisol (the stress hormone) and lower levels of serotonin (the feel-good hormone).

Biologically speaking, the body responds to stress by activating the sympathetic nervous system, which is responsible for producing the fight-or-flight response. This physiological reaction involves an increase in heart rate and respiration as well as a decrease in digestion and other processes. This response can be beneficial in certain situations, such as when one needs to quickly respond to a threat. However, when this response is activated too often or when it is not needed, it can lead to physical and mental health problems.

Additionally, research has shown that the immune system can be affected by anxiety disorders as well. Those with anxiety may have higher levels of inflammation in their bodies, which can lead to a decrease in overall health and an increase in vulnerability to disease. Therefore, proper treatment for an anxiety disorder is an important step in improving overall health and wellbeing.

By understanding the causes of anxiety disorders,

we can help to develop better treatment plans and strategies for those living with them. Through proper diagnosis, lifestyle changes, self-care strategies, and professional help from a mental health provider, anxiety disorders can be managed effectively.

Eating Disorders

Eating disorders are a complex mental health issue that is defined by an unhealthy relationship with food. It can manifest in many ways, including binge eating, purging, or severe restriction of food intake. Eating disorders involve more than just physical symptoms; they also have psychological components that affect people's relationships, their view of themselves, and their overall sense of wellbeing.

There are many potential causes of eating disorders, including biological factors, environmental influences, and psychological aspects. Biological factors such as hormone imbalances or genetic predisposition can lead to the development of an eating disorder. Environmental influences, such as negative body image due to social media pressures or restrictive diets prescribed by a loved one, can also contribute to the development of an eating disorder. Finally, psychological issues such as a traumatic childhood experience or low self-esteem can cause someone to develop an unhealthy relationship with food.

Eating Disorders Pathophysiology

The pathophysiology of eating disorders is complex and involves many different factors. An understanding of the biological, environmental, and psychological components that contribute to these conditions can help inform treatment plans and support individuals in their recovery journey.

Biological factors may play a role in the development of an eating disorder, particularly genetics or chemical imbalances in the body. Studies have shown that hormonal dysregulation, particularly related to the hormones leptin and ghrelin, can lead to changes in appetite or food cravings.

Environmental influences also play an important role in eating disorders. Social media has a large impact on how people perceive their bodies, with images of thinness portrayed as the ideal body type. Societal pressure to 'look a certain way' can contribute to unhealthy eating habits. Additionally, trauma or an unstable home environment can lead to the development of eating disorders.

Finally, psychological issues such as depression, anxiety, and low self-esteem are strongly linked with the onset of an eating disorder. Anxiety in particular has been found to be a risk factor for developing an eating disorder due to its restrictive effects on eating habits. Additionally, individuals with low self-esteem may use food as a way to cope with difficult emotions or try to take control over their life.

Treatment for an eating disorder should be tailored to each individual, taking into account the biological, environmental, and psychological factors that are contributing to their condition. Cognitive-behavioral therapy (CBT) can be effective in helping individuals understand the underlying issues that are driving their behavior, and help them to develop more positive coping strategies. Additionally, medical monitoring and dietary advice may be necessary to ensure that physical health is maintained.

CONCLUSION

Pathophysiology is a complex field of study that encompasses many different concepts and approaches. By understanding the fundamentals of pathophysiology, healthcare professionals can better diagnose and treat diseases and medical conditions, as well as influence public health outcomes. As new technologies continue to develop, it is important for medical practitioners to stay up-to-date on the latest research in order to provide quality care for their patients.

Key concepts of Pathophysiology :

1. Homeostasis: This is the process of maintaining a dynamic equilibrium in the body's internal environment, even with changes that occur in external conditions. Homeostasis is regulated by feedback mechanisms that detect and respond to any deviation from normal levels.

2. Pathogenesis: This refers to the origin and development of a disease or medical condition. It involves both genetic and environmental factors and can include the body's own immune response to an infection.

3. Etiology: This refers to the cause of a disease or medical condition, including both internal and external factors that contribute to its development.

4. Morbidity: This term is used to describe the severity of a disease or medical condition, generally in terms of its symptoms and how it affects the quality of life.

5. Prognosis: This term is used to describe a medical condition's expected outcome, including its potential complications, as well as any treatments that may be necessary for recovery.

6. Epidemiology: This is the study of disease patterns in populations, which can help identify risk factors and develop preventive measures for certain diseases or medical conditions.

7. Comorbidity: This refers to the co-occurrence of two or more illnesses in a patient, which can complicate diagnosis and treatment.

8. Syndromes: This term refers to clusters of signs and symptoms that are indicative of specific diseases or medical conditions, providing clues that may help with diagnosis and treatment.

9. Pharmacotherapy: This is the use of medications to treat a disease or medical condition, either alone or in combination with other treatments such as therapy or surgery.

The understanding of pathophysiology has come

a long way in modern medicine. By studying the various mechanisms that cause disease, we can better equip ourselves to prevent and treat diseases. From deciphering the body's response to tissue injury to uncovering the intricacies of how particular drugs act on cells, pathophysiology is an important part of healthcare today. Through a deeper understanding of pathology and its underlying processes, physicians can enhance patient care by providing more personalized treatments and improved outcomes.

In addition to being used in clinical practice, pathophysiology is also used in research to investigate the cause of diseases and develop new treatments. By studying how cells respond to certain stressors or medications, researchers are able to gain valuable insights into potential therapeutic targets for disease. Furthermore, by studying the way diseases progress and spread through populations, researchers can better understand how to prevent them from occurring in the first place.

Pathophysiology is an important part of medicine that has a strong influence on healthcare decisions today. Through research and clinical practice, physicians are able to use this information to develop more effective treatments and provide better outcomes for their patients. Pathophysiology plays a key role in both the diagnosis and treatment of diseases, so it is essential to continue researching this field in order to advance medical care into the future.

At its core, pathophysiology is about understanding disease processes and how they interact with other systems within the body. By studying these various components, we can better understand how diseases progress and develop strategies for treatment and prevention. Through this continuing research, we will be able to create more effective treatments and improve the overall quality of life for patients around the world.

The study of pathophysiology is only going to become more important as time goes on. With the continued development of medical technology and techniques, it is essential that we stay on top of the latest advancements in order to take advantage of them. By taking a deeper dive into the complexities of disease processes, we can arm ourselves with the knowledge needed to help prevent and treat diseases effectively.

By uncovering the mysteries behind pathophysiology, healthcare providers can use this knowledge to improve patient care and ensure that individuals are receiving the best possible treatments. Armed with this understanding, we can continue to make advances in medical technology and increase the quality of life for patients around the world. Through research and clinical practice, pathophysiology will remain a cornerstone of modern medicine for years to come.

Further exploration into pathophysiology can lead to new insights into disease processes, treatments, and preventative strategies. By continuing to study how diseases develop and progress, we can help empower medical professionals with the knowledge they need to make informed decisions about patient care. With this understanding of pathology, physicians can provide more comprehensive and effective treatments for a variety of illnesses. As our knowledge continues to grow in this field, it is important to stay at the forefront of medical research and practice in order to ensure that every patient receives the best possible care.

MAY I ASK YOU FOR A
SMALL FAVOR?

Before you go, please I need your assistance! In case you like this book, might you be able to please share your opinion on Amazon and compose a legit review? It will take only one moment for you, yet be an extraordinary favour for me. Since I'm not a famous writer and I don't have a large distributing organization supporting me. I read each and every review and hop around with happiness like a little child each time my audience remarks on my books and gives me their fair criticism! ☺. In case you didn't appreciate the book or had an issue with it, kindly get in touch with me via email D.beckology@gmail.com and reveal to me how I can improve it.

Made in United States
Troutdale, OR
10/21/2024

23968539R00105